The Handbook of
HOSPICE
CARE

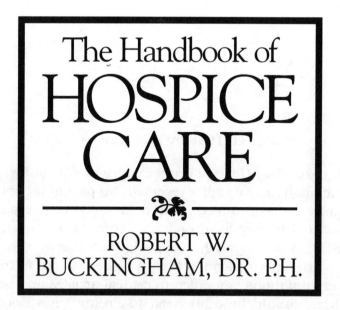

The Handbook of
HOSPICE
CARE

ROBERT W.
BUCKINGHAM, DR. P.H.

With A Foreword By
ROSEMARY JOHNSON HURZELER
CHAIRMAN, HOSPICE ASSOCIATION OF AMERICA

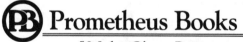

Prometheus Books

59 John Glenn Drive
Amherst, New York 14228-2197

Published 1996 by Prometheus Books

00 99 98 97 96   5 4 3 2 1

Library of Congress Cataloging-in-Publication Data

Buckingham, Robert W.
    The handbook of hospice care / Robert W. Buckingham.
        p.   cm.
    Includes bibliographical references.
    ISBN 1-57392-060-6 (paper : alk. paper)
    1. Hospice care. 2. Hospices (Terminal care)—United
States. I. Title.
R726.8.B824   1996
362.1′75—dc20   96–11357
                                                 CIP

Printed in the United States of America on acid-free paper

to H.L.S.
my love
my inspiration
my teammate

Contents

Acknowledgments

I must sincerely thank two wonderful women for their work on this book. The first is Ms. Kate Mahoney, for her wonderful chapter on contemporary issues in hospice care and her work in putting this manuscript together. Her persistence and dedication to the hospice concept of care is greatly appreciated.

I would also like to thank Ms. Kathy McGuinness for her relentless effort in editing this book. Ms. McGuinness is certainly the treasure of Prometheus.

This book would not exist without the commitment of Editor-in-Chief Steven Mitchell and the friendship and advice of Mr. Dan Wasinger, also of Prometheus. These two men are the backbone of Prometheus Books and I salute them.

Dr. Robert W. Buckingham

Foreword

The end of life is a dimension that can never be known until we experience it ourselves. To live life until the very end in comfort and with the right support illustrates the quality of the society in which we live. In *The Handbook of Hospice Care*, Robert Buckingham examines the truths and explains the "what ifs" about the end of life, describing the solid care and support available through hospice for those who need it.

This book, a welcome addition to the body of hospice-related literature, is a wonderful way to share the hospice message. In the seemingly small community of hospice providers around the country, everyone who contributes is a friend. Dr. Buckingham's work has helped to keep hospice on the minds and lips of professionals and lay persons alike. As a Fellow in the John D.

Thompson Hospice Institute for Education, Training, and Research, the teaching arm of The Connecticut Hospice, Inc., Robert Buckingham is committed to educating his colleagues and the community about hospice care. Dr. Buckingham became acquainted with hospice care over two decades ago as the Director of Research at The Connecticut Hospice, Inc., the first hospice in the United States. It is only fitting that as we head into the next millennium, Dr. Buckingham is on the forefront of hospice research.

Those of us who are enmeshed in the particulars of hospice care look eagerly toward its future. As medical practices improve and society changes we must change with it. Hospice programs can now care for any disease, for patients of any age, including children, and can incorporate all types of family situations into the plan of care. We look to a future without labels when this type of care, which addresses various aspects of patients and their lives, becomes universally acceptable and accessible. Having inspired a generation with his previous works on hospice care, Dr. Buckingham's current research and this book will hopefully serve to inspire those who will provide hospice care in the future. This work envisions a health-care continuum that would embrace state of the art hospice and palliative care. To see the concepts and practice of hospice care woven into the academic and clinical settings would be a great accomplishment for those, like Dr. Buckingham, who have devoted so much time and energy to exploring and improving care.

Our hospice patients leave us a legacy of choices made and needs expressed. Hospice means quality of life for as long as life lasts. Dr. Buckingham's work will support all those who seek to create opportunities for compassion and choice so that the end of life can celebrate those who have lived life and those who have loved them.

* * *

Rosemary Johnson Hurzeler, R.N., M.P.H., H.A., is the President and CEO of The Connecticut Hospice, Inc., the first American hospice, and the John D. Thompson Hospice Institute for Education, Training, and Research. Ms. Johnson Hurzeler is currently the Chairman of the Hospice Association of America.

Prologue

Introductory Thoughts
from Dr. Robert Buckingham

Dying is part of the process of living. As a leaf buds and shines its youthful color, it must also mature, die, and decay. We are all leaves on the tree of life, and we all must fall someday. We should not fear death, nor should we ignore it. We must not protect ourselves from the reality of the end of our physical being. We should instead be concerned about living each and every day as fully as possible.

Unfortunately, the issue of death has been denied, hidden, and thus feared by our society. Many physicians, even, are strangers to the real issues of dying. Historically, physicians have been taught to diagnose, treat, and cure. They look at death as failure and therefore shy away from those dying patients whom they believe they have "failed." Although recent attempts by a few lay people have brought the important issue of death into people's consciousness, more efforts must be made to educate the medical community as well as the public about the importance of hospice care and its philosophy of allowing one to live the last stages of life with dignity.

This book attempts to familiarize the reader with the basic concepts of hospice care as a philosophy whose time has come. It incorporates pain control, symptom control (physical and psychological), continuous medical and nursing accessibility, medical direction, utilization of volunteers, home care, training of family members as care givers, and a bereavement program for the survivors.

In 1970, my fifty-year-old mother (a New York City fashion designer) was dying of breast cancer. She was cared for in a prestigious teaching institution which offered good general care but poor palliative care. The staff was not trained to ease pain without curing the ailment. There were no hospices then. No one talked to me; no one talked to my father or sister. We had many questions, but no one to address them to. My mother lingered in discomfort. Death was a release for her, which I do not regret, but I regret the way she died. Many of her medical, nursing, and emotional needs were never addressed. While traditional approaches to health care emphasize cure and the prolongation of life, such care is restrictive and insensitive to the needs of the terminal patient and the family who have accepted the reality of death and wish to focus on the quality of life remaining.

In the early 1970s I was a graduate student in the Yale School of Medicine. Unbeknown to me at that time, an interdisciplinary faculty committee was meeting weekly at Yale, arranging to bring over from England a new concept and philosophy of medical and nursing care—hospice care. It was designed for people with a very limited prognosis (six months or less to live), and encompassed psychological, spiritual, and medical problems. Upon completion of my doctoral work at Yale, the dean of the Yale Nursing School asked if I would be interested in working as director of research at the first and only developing hospice in the United States. I took the position, and it enabled me to interview and study many wonderful patients who, like my mother, were suffering from end-stage disease. These patients and their families taught me the meaning of life. I realized that through the eyes of the dying one can realize the significant issues of living.

The early days of the New Haven hospice were very taxing to the staff. We suffered many setbacks and defeats. Educating the medical community was the most difficult task of all, and it still is. Without the support of the National Cancer Institute, the hospice concept of care in the United States would not have survived. In those years we proved to Washington and the American people that hospice care was needed in the United States. Since 1976, more than eight hundred hospices have been developed nationwide. I am happy to report that hospice care is now reimbursable under Medicare/Medicaid and private insurance companies like Blue Cross and Blue Shield. We have proved that hospice care is often better than traditional acute-care facilities and considerably less expensive.

Historically—since the industrial revolution—dying has been a coming-apart experience for most families. Hospice care concentrates on making the process of dying a *coming-together* experience for patient and family. Hospice is not a place or an institution but a philosophy of care in which the person is considered of primary importance and the disease is secondary. For the last eighteen years, I have spent my academic career developing, managing, researching, and teaching about the hospice concept of care. It is my lifelong wish to have the word "hospice" disappear and the concept and philosophy of hospice care prevail with all medical, nursing, and allied health professionals.

My years of research into the hospice concept have brought me to the belief that in order to live the way you choose, you must be assertive. That applies to how you die, as well. Many people are more content to be regulated by others than to take charge of their own lives. Epictetus wrote of freedom in his *Discourses*: "No man is free who is not master of himself." Freedom to choose the way we live and die is what families and patients must strive for.

This is my tenth book. As a professor of public health for eighteen years, I write this book for those of you with an interest or concern for people who are terminally ill. Working with terminally ill cancer and AIDS patients for many years, I have obtained much wisdom from them, wisdom that I would like to share with you. The following "Lessons from Dr. Buckingham" are lessons from my patient-teachers on which I lecture frequently. They were previously published in *Among Friends: Hospice Care for the Person with AIDS*,* but their message is equally as important for this book.

*Robert W. Buckingham (Amherst, N.Y.: Prometheus Books, 1992).

Lesson No. 1: *Keep your life simple.* Many people have a tendency to complicate their lives with trivial matters and pursuits. It is very important to look at your life and not get wrapped up with insignificant trivia. Be able to focus on what really is important. What are your interests? What are your loves? Don't worry about things that you cannot change. Worry about the things that you can change.

Lesson No. 2: *Ask yourself three basic questions.* I have stated often to my medical and undergraduate students that there are three basic questions that we must ask ourselves. They are: (1) Who am I? (2) What do I want? and (3) Where do I want to go? At different times in our lives, we will have different answers to these questions, but the answers are not as important as remembering to ask the questions.

Lesson No. 3: *Eliminate the disadvantage complex.* The disadvantage complex is something that people say to themselves, subconsciously or consciously, like, "I'm too old," "I'm not smart enough," "I'm not attractive enough," or "I'm too fat." No one is too old, we are all of basically equal intelligence, and attraction is broad. We must not compare ourselves to others.

Lesson No. 4: *Challenge yourself.* It is important that we all try at times to challenge ourselves. For us to become stronger, to face another day, we must not become complacent with our being. Without our self-challenge there is no growth. So many Americans are content to sit by their television set and to be entertained into a state of lethargy. There is so much going on outside our windows: so much to do, to see, and to feel. We must not be afraid of the challenge presented by new opportunities.

Lesson No. 5: *Do not compare yourself to others.* As I said earlier, it is very difficult to go on with our lives, to make them fruitful, if we are always comparing ourselves to others. It is a simple lesson: you are special. As you know, we can't compare oranges to apples; every human is different. Many of us are brought up with our parents always telling us things like, "Oh, I wish you could be as smart as Johnny" or "I wish you could be as polite as little Suzy." It is a wrong lesson to learn. Take pride in your uniqueness. Do not be afraid to be who you are.

Lesson No. 6: *Maintain a positive outlook.* In life there are three kinds of people: those who say, "Things are going to be okay"; those who say, "Things are not going to be okay"; and those who say, "Whatever will be will be." We want to be the people for whom everything will be okay. Positive thoughts will become affirmations of our being; without them we cannot affirm the glory of our being or our becoming.

Lesson No. 7: *Stop complaining.* As a university professor for all these years, I have listened to students complaining every day: "This class is boring," "This professor is boring," "My boss doesn't care; he/she does not treat me nicely." If we listen to those around us, we will always hear people complaining. These are people, I think, who are focused on the minus signs of life, and who like to wallow in their own self-pity and negativism. They are slowly digging a hole for themselves. Don't fall into this trap. Stop complaining. When you have problems—and we all do—it is important for us to look up and say, very simply, "It will pass."

Lesson No. 8: *Be here now.* This is one great lesson I have learned from my patients who face the challenges of cancer and AIDS. It, too, is a simple lesson. Today is our most precious possession. Do not look back fondly to memories of yesterday or ahead to the possibilities of tomorrow; focus on the importance of becoming today, being today, being here now. Remember, life is only so long. No matter how long it is, it is never long enough. In one of my books, I stated, "The greatest tragedy in life is not that we are going to die; the greatest tragedy in life is not living life fully." Now is the time on which to focus. Be here now. Enjoy every moment you have.

Lesson No. 9: *You are responsible for your own happiness.* Do not expect others to bring it to you. Again, the ability to be content and happy lies with ourselves. It is a matter of self-responsibility, of internal signals and not external feedback.

Lesson No. 10: *Keep the craziness in you alive.* I like this lesson. Simply stated, don't lose touch with the craziness in you. All of us walk the fine line between normality and acceptance on the one hand, and, on the other, the little "crazy" thoughts we have. These thoughts might sometimes seem immature, silly, or insignificant. Sometimes they become actions. It's okay to be a little crazy, to laugh at yourself and the world. Keep this craziness alive in yourself. Wallow in it. It's fun. Remember, life is meant to be enjoyed. It's not serious business all the time.

Lesson No. 11: *Let go of your anger, hurt, or pain.* I have learned this lesson with my patients' families. Do not hold on to anger, hurt, or pain. They will only take away your energy for loving life. Don't let your anger and pain stay inside you very long. Deal with them, speak about them, but don't be afraid to let them go.

Lesson No. 12: *Adventure through your life.* This is probably the most important lesson. It is vital that we look at life as an adventure, no matter how long we have. There are so many wonderful things that we can do, so many wonderful people we can touch and love. The greatest adventure in life is loving and enjoying other people.

I would like to go on now with a few more lessons I have learned from my patient-teachers. They have taught me to understand what love is. Quite simply, they have taught me that to love successfully you must live your life the way you choose. By that I mean you must be able to stand up for your beliefs; you must not be monitored by the dictates and beliefs of others. Many of us handicap ourselves by a lack of self-confidence. But we must draw strength from ourselves and not let other people victimize us. You see so many people in America today who seem content just being regulated by others. They don't want to take charge of their own lives.

You must say, "This is my life. I choose to be happy. I choose to be depressed. I choose to be sad. I choose to be positive. I choose to be in love. I choose to be without love. I choose to be strong. I choose to succeed. I choose to be weak. I choose to fail." We might victimize ourselves because we've convinced ourselves that some people won't like us or that disaster is around the corner. Be careful of these thoughts. They can take away your effectiveness and future success. Thoughts like this will betray your internal support system. The bravest thing you can do when you have thoughts like these is to profess courage and act accordingly. In what I call the professing of courage, I am referring to statements like, "I can do it." "I will be liked." "I will be accepted." " I am strong." You must remove and eliminate the disadvantage complex.

Another word of advice—stay away from people who want you to join them in their misery. So many depressed and sad souls are only looking for others on whom they can unload their baggage. Remember, these people can zap your courage.

Another lesson I have learned from people who have a dreadful disease and a short time to live is that we should not victimize others. By this I am referring to making such statements as, "I don't understand why you say those things." "How could anyone with your brains and background do such a thing?" "Do it for me." "You've offended me." "I demand an apology." Avoid making such victimizing statements. They will not help your relationships with others. And never place loyalty to institutions and things above loyalty to yourself. Remember, as Shakespeare wrote in the first act of *Hamlet*, "This above all, to thine own self be true, and it must follow, as the night the day, thou canst not then be false to any man."[1]

Remember that life is a continuous series of experiences rather than one single experience. I believe that our successes can only be measured by our constant motivation, perseverance, and a number of failures. I believe we must fail in order to succeed. Remember, for us to live fully we must learn to use things and to love people, not love things and use people.

In closing, I would like to make a very simple com-

---

1. *Hamlet*, 5.34.75.

ment about life itself. Humankind, unlike the other animals, has either forgotten or has never learned that the sole purpose of life is to enjoy it. We must reach out, touch it, enjoy it, live it, and love it. Again, we must look at the opportunities that we have today, Make today count and don't ever forget to count your blessings.

FURTHER THOUGHTS FROM DR. BUCKINGHAM

1. You are never given a dream without the power of making it come true.

2. Listen to your heart. It is sometimes wiser than your mind.

3. The happenings of life are there because you have drawn them there.

4. Find your cause; make it yours.

5. Life is more of a comedy than a tragedy.

6. A monarch butterfly has only moments but has time enough.

7. True love is like a cactus, a plant of slow growth; it must withstand the summer monsoon of clouds, wind, and rain before it blooms its wondrous flower.

8. Compassion is what unites people; opinions are what separate them.

9. Be cautious in choosing a lover, more cautious in letting one go.

10. Most people build walls around themselves; after they occupy them for a while, they become comfortable with the walls and feel secure in their little prison. After a while they abandon hope of ever doing more with their lives. Many begin to suffer living deaths.

11. Think positively. Reading or saying a thought over and over in our mind will eventually imprint the thought, and thought can become reality.

12. Accept responsibility for your own feelings but not for the feelings and actions of others.

13. Today is the day to tell someone you love him or her. This is a day to live fully in the moment.

14. Making mistakes is natural—self-forgiveness is more difficult but absolutely necessary.

15. Stand up and go forward. Get off the couch of life.

16. Yesterday is gone and is history. Let it go. Take spirit in the new dawn. Make it happy and fulfilling.

17. Falling back is part of moving forward.

18. Do not let old relationships hold you back from personal growth.

19. Happiness comes from being happy with what we already have and expressing gratitude to God for it.

20. Do not search for joy. It is within you.

1

Hospice Philosophy of Care

Even though more than twenty years have passed since hospice care was introduced to the United States, the general lay population still lacks a comprehensive view of its basic concepts. I have written this book to remedy this situation, interweaving the philosophy of hospice throughout. This book is best suited for the person or persons who are about to face the loss of a loved one and would like to explore the possibility of choosing hospice care over other types of care. Intended readers include, but are not limited to, lay audiences, entry level hospice professionals, and health care professionals who are contemplating entering the hospice arena.

Chapters 1 and 2 will give the reader an overview of the philosophy and history of hospice care. Contemporary hospice issues are discussed in chapter 3. In chapter 4, the administrative aspect of hospice is explored along with a breakdown of the hospice structure and its components. Chapters 6 and 7 focus on two target populations for hospice care: children and persons with AIDS. Grief management is discussed in chapter 8. Hints on how to start a hospice program in your community follow, and the book ends by projecting into the future of hospice.

DEFINITION

Hospice is primarily a philosophy of care and a program for the terminally ill. It is not necessarily a facility. The program can be carried out in the patient's home, in a separate freestanding facility, in a department of a general, acute-care hospital, or as a separate facility attached either physically or organizationally to a general hospital.[1] The hospice approach centers on helping the dying and their loved ones to maintain the dignity and humaness of the dying process and providing sophisticated medical and nursing care. The focus of the hospice approach and philosophy is to help the dying to live as fully as possible during the time that remains. Through the control of symptoms, hospice care seeks to eliminate the suffering that accompanies the dying process.[2]

Hospice care, however, goes beyond the elimination of symptoms. The focus is not on the disease itself, but on the patient and family. The hospice community makes every effort to provide appropriate care and to promote a caring community which is sensitive to the needs of the patients and families. It is hoped that this will help them attain a degree of mental and spiritual preparedness for death.

PALLIATIVE CARE VERSUS CURATIVE CARE

The health system is oriented toward the cure of disease. Physicians are taught to diagnose and treat disease with the expectation of cure as a consequence. This orientation ignores the fuller definition of medical care dating back to the fifteenth century which is to cure sometimes, to relieve often, and to comfort always.[3] The cure of disease is not the goal of all medical therapy. Seen from a broader and more complete perspective, the goal of medical therapy is the provision of suitable treatment to the patient. Treatment is appropriate if the physician applies one of two complementary systems at the correct time. The first is concerned with eliminating a controllable disease and the second with relieving the symptoms of an incurable illness. When cure is not possible, improving the quality of life of the patient through palliative care is the appropriate approach.[4] It is important to stress that palliative care does not simply mean the mitigation of suffering by symptom relief alone; it includes everything that hospice does to help the patient continue life in as near to a usual manner as possible. This means helping the patient and the family make the best use of the time they have left to share.[5]

THE GOALS OF HOSPICE

In a general hospital, the staff works toward attaining four basic goals: investigation, diagnosis, cure, and the prolongation of life. These goals are cumulative; each builds on the former and the first three goals must be successfully attained for the fourth goal, the prolongation of life, to be reached. Through testing and analysis (investigation), the medical staff determines (diagnoses) the cause of the problem, allowing them to create a treatment plan that will eradicate (cure) the disease, thereby prolonging the patient's life.

The goals of hospice, however, are quite different and may be reached independently of each other. Hospices seek to provide relief from the distressing symptoms of the disease, provide sustained expert care, provide the security of a caring environment, and provide the assurance that patients and their families will not be abandoned.[6]

Symptom control is a major ingredient of hospice care. After physicians and nurses determine the cause of the symptoms, attempts are made to apply treatment that will alleviate them and avoid unnecessary side effects. Because the competent hospice team is aware that the terminally ill patient has extremely low physical, physiological, and emotional reserves, the entire team, which includes the patient and family, chooses a treatment that will not complicate patient management. Every effort is made to prevent symptoms by applying appropriate therapies at intervals that maintain a continuing beneficial effect. Finally, symptom control demands continuous monitoring of the patient. This allows for immediate and proper modification of care by responding to changes in the patient's condition.[7]

Hospice provides sustained expert care available around the clock, whenever the patient might require assistance, regardless of location. Families are able to keep their relative at home due to the twenty-four-hour service available through hospices. Care is provided by an expert team whose members include the physician, nurses, social workers, the family, and trained volunteers. The patient's entire spectrum of needs (physical, intellectual, emotional, social, financial, and spiritual) is addressed. Causes of happiness and distress for the patient and family are of concern to the hospice team.[8] This caring environment is essential to the hospice approach.

The greatest fear of those who are terminally ill is not death and pain, but the fear of being left alone and dying without anyone by their side. Hospice provides the patients and the families with the assurance that they will not be abandoned, and thus, helps alleviate one of the major problems of terminally ill patients. Emotional support is an essential aspect of hospice care.[9] The emphasis is on making the process of dying a *coming-together* experience for the patient and family. Even after death has occurred, emotional support for the surviving family members continues. This may include individual bereavement support, follow-up visits by hospice staff, and bereavement groups.

THE HOSPICE TEAM

Care is provided for the terminally ill patient by a multidisciplinary patient care team comprised of everyone who participates in the patient's care: physicians, nurses, social workers, physical therapists, pharmacologists, chaplains, volunteers, patients, and families. Because hospice care is personal, the team is shaped by the personal needs and preferences of each patient and family. The team meets together at least weekly to review the patient's and family's progress. These meetings provide the team members with an opportunity to share their perspectives regarding both assessment and management of the patient's symptoms. Issues that may be discussed are specifics of medical and nursing care; pain control; effects of illness such as dry mouth and anorexia; and social issues involving the family, including denial. Other issues may include strategies by which the primary care person can cope with exhaustion and the need for support. This kind of teamwork enables each member to approach the patient and the family with a personal, hands-on understanding as well as a professional understanding of all aspects of care. This cooperative approach allows hospice to provide its patients and loved ones with a comprehensive program of care, and at the same time enables the team members to cope with the stress that is intrinsic to working with the grief and suffering of others.[10] Each team member plays an important and active role in caring for the patient. The roles of the physician, nurse, and volunteers will be described in more detail.

Physicians

Physicians play a pivotal and crucial role in the program. First of all, they have a responsibility and authority, both professional and legal, which no other hospice team member has. Physicians order diagnostic studies and establish a valid diagnosis. They are also the only member of the team who have a license to prescribe medications that provide the most effective palliative care. Doctors also certify legal death and secure reimbursement for ancillary health care services (supportive health services that utilize allied physicians). The team looks to the physicians for assurance that it has satisfied its responsibilities in a medically competent and effective manner. The doctors guide program administration so that hospices meet the needs of their patients and the families.[11]

Although hospices have their own physicians on staff, the referring doctor is encouraged to remain a part of the patient's program of care after the referral to hospice has been made. Some doctors choose to relinquish control of their patient entirely, while others opt to become a part of the hospice team.

Nurses

In most home health agencies or hospice programs, it is the nurse who assesses the patient's physical condition, provides interventions, and discusses with the physician relevant changes in the patient. Other responsibilities include teaching team members about infection control, pain and symptom management, and comfort measures. In the case of a person with AIDS, because the course of AIDS is so unpredictable, a nurse must be on call twenty-four hours per day.[12]

What the nurse offers depends largely on the condition of the patient, the particular symptoms present in the illness, and the existing degree of independence. This care involves not only symptom and pain control, but also such items as bathing, control of odor, mouth care, care of hair, as well as bowel and bladder care. Depending on the setting, the nurse may take direct charge of some of these services, or they may be provided by attendants or volunteers. The nurse has the responsibility of caring for and closely observing the patient. Patients have to be taught to say when they are in pain or discomfort, but the nurse must be able to anticipate pain and thus keep the patient as pain free as possible.[13] Hospice nurses work within physicians' prescription guidelines for dose ranges and flexible intervals to effectively and safely adjust the amount and frequency of pain medications for patients who have prolonged, variable, and sometimes severe pain.[14]

Volunteers

Volunteers play a large role in bringing about the high level of personal care found in hospices. They are carefully interviewed, trained, and screened before being placed on a hospice team. Listening and communication skills are primary, along with an understanding of the

humane philosophies that are fundamental to the program. Other skills that are essential to a hospice volunteer are an enthusiasm to work with people who need
understanding and guidance at home, a love for others,
and a desire to help. When technical skills are needed,
they are covered in volunteer training.

Volunteers may serve in a variety of positions: direct
care givers, receptionists, public speakers, photogra-
phers, writers, or researchers. A good volunteer gets to
know the patient and family and become a friend, which
may be one of the most important functions that person
could perform. The patient and family often need the
support and relief that volunteers can offer. Many times
it is easier for the patient and family to relate to and
confide in volunteers than it is for them to deal with a
professional. Also, when a relationship develops during
an illness, the volunteers may become an important vis-
itor during bereavement, when their most important
role entails listening and offering compassion and understanding to the family. Volunteers can report social
problems such as any increase in the use of alcohol or
barbiturates by those grieving. They can help with tasks
like emptying closets of the deceased, getting a lawyer,
and funeral arrangements. But most important,
throughout the illness they offer friendly interaction to
the patient and family.

Volunteers bring fresh outlooks to hospice and provide energy and support that the program needs in
order to exist. Although volunteers do not replace paid
staff, they do supplement hospice services and provide
needed support to the patient, the family, and other
team members. The volunteer does not receive pay and

usually is not a health professional (doctor, nurse, or social worker). Volunteers are important members of the team and largely contribute to making hospice a caring community.

By participating in a hospice program, each team member will have the opportunity to learn from the other members, each of whom brings special perspectives to the program. For a hospice program to be effective, there must be intense internal communication, both professionally and personally, among all team members.

BEREAVEMENT SERVICES

Because hospice views the unit of care as including both the patient and the family, bereavement programs are integral to the concepts underlying this philosophy of care. The overwhelming evidence of the suffering and adjustments families must make after a loved one's death clearly indicate the need for ongoing care for the survivors. The hospice concept of treating the patient and family as the unit of care is not only humane but very practical socially. Grief, unassisted and unprepared for, can lead to delinquency of children, divorce, drug and alcohol abuse, and poor physical health.

Preparation for bereavement, which is usually an aspect of hospice care, includes preparing the will, discussing the funeral, and planning for the future. The patient and his family help each other face the inevitable. Furthermore, the closeness established between patient and family during a peaceful terminal phase can ease acceptance of death. Survivors are likely to feel less, if any, guilt, and to have little, if any, unfinished business.

After the death of a loved one, hospice bereavement programs help survivors cope with their feelings of grief and loss through discussion groups, follow-up visits, and other types of programming. When it appears that the mourning period may extend beyond a reasonable period, hospice volunteers are able to recommend appropriate measures to avoid any unhealthy behavior patterns which may develop among the survivors.

INSTITUTIONALLY BASED HOSPICES COMPARED TO INDEPENDENT HOSPICES

Institutionally based hospices usually consist of a wing in a hospital with a six-bed unit. An independent hospice, on the other hand, has no affiliation with a hospital; it stands alone. It has been estimated that fewer than 20 percent of the hospices which currently exist are wholly independent although the majority are free-standing (i.e., they are not physically located within an acute-care hospital). Most hospices, however, are affiliated with one or more hospitals. Sometimes the two types of hospice complement each other and at other times they compete. Institutionally based hospices are often excellent due to the dedication of the medical directors and other staff, but there are some matters that trouble those who are involved in hospice development. Hospices housed in acute-care hospitals have significantly higher rates of institutional deaths than home-care hospices with inpatient backup. Patients of a hospital-based hospice unit die more frequently in the inpatient unit than at home. Home-care options in institutionally based hospices must be strengthened to be sure that patients receive a real choice. The institutional setting can become self-perpetuating, and administrators of such hospices must be sure that patients are not institutionalized unnecessarily. Home care should always be the focus, and hospice inpatient units should serve only as backup. Ideally, even if the inpatient unit is necessary temporarily, with additional support the patient may be able to return home. There is concern that higher rates of institutional deaths in institutionally based hospices reflect a loss of hospice philosophy. If we are not vigilant about maintaining hospice standards of care, we could end up right where we started, with inappropriate care for the terminally ill.

Institutional hospices in the acute-care setting are surrounded by an atmosphere of urgency, haste, and machinery. Hospital administrators often feel financial pressure to fill empty beds, and it may be that this pressure extends to hospices in hospitals. There may also be a temptation to fill beds in other hospital areas with "hospice" patients, and hospice medical directors may find themselves struggling to maintain the psychological and physical environment necessary for hospice patients. The results may be unsatisfactory not only for the patient, but for the medical director and for the hospital administration as well.

Sir Michael Sobell House in Oxford, England, is a hospice established as a separate unit located on the grounds of Churchill Hospital. Sandol Stoddard, a journalist who wrote an early book promoting hospice, describes Sobell House as homey and cozy, with the characteristics of a small community. Children are welcomed with treats and decorations designed for them. Stoddard says: "Everything about the unit suggests medical expertise, yet nothing here is strange, forbidding, or frightening."[15]

Hospices within a hospital do not have as much freedom to create a homey environment, and usually do not have as much space as an independent hospice. The playschools one sees at St. Christopher's (a hospice in London, England, which can be considered the first modern hospice), or at The Connecticut Hospice, Inc., in Branford, Connecticut, are absent. The atmosphere and visiting hours in an institutionally based hospice are more likely to be restrictive for children. Hospices within an institution have a more hospital-like environment, although the care for terminally ill patients is superior to the hospitals and more personalized. Institutionally based hospices hope that the hospital climate will be modified and improved as other areas of the hospital see the success of hospice methods. Hospices within institutions may serve as models and teachers if care is taken to adhere to hospice philosophy.

NOTES

1. K. Cohen, *Hospice, Prescription for Terminal Care* (Germantown, Md.: Aspen Systems Corp., 1979), pp. 2–4.

2. D. McKell, "Hospice Care: A New Concept for the Care of the Terminally Ill and Their Families," workshop at UCLA Extension, Los Angeles, April 1978.

3. C. Corr and D. Corr, *Hospice Care: Principles and Practice* (New York: Springer Publishing, 1983), pp. 104–105.

4. D. Shepard, "Principles and Practice of Palliative Care," *Canadian Medical Association Journal* 116 (1977): 525–26.

5. Ibid.

6. Cohen, *Hospice, Prescription for Terminal Care.*

7. Ibid.

8. Corr and Corr, *Hospice Care.*

9. Ibid.

10. Ibid.

11. Ibid. and W. Bulkin and H. Lukashok, "Rx for the Dying: The Case for Hospice," *New England Journal of Medicine* 318, no. 6 (1988): 316–78.

12. J. Martin, "Hospice and Home Care for Persons with AIDS/ARC," *Death Studies* 12 (1988): 468–69.

13. Corr and Corr, *Hospice Care.*

14. M. McCaffery, "Pain Management: Nurses Lead the Way to New Priorities," *American Journal of Nursing* 90 (1990): 45–46.

15. Sandol Stoddard, *The Hospice Movement* (New York: Stein & Day, 1978), pp. 40–142.

2

Hospice Then . . . Hospice Now

THE HISTORY OF HOSPICE

"Hospitality," "hospitable," "host," "hostess," "hospital," "hostel," "hotel," "hospice": all these words have the same root, the Latin word *hospes*. All include the ideas of kindness and generosity to strangers or caring for our fellow beings and offering them nourishment and refreshment.

Ancient hospices or hospitals (the two were one for a number of centuries) provided sanctuary for the poor wayfarer, the sick and dying, the woman in labor, the orphan, the needy, and the religious pilgrim. Medieval hospices were generally run by religious orders, serving the Lord by serving His poor, His sick, and those in need of shelter. Welcome was extended by hospices throughout Europe in major towns and cities, in villages, in remote monastic hermitages, and along the route to the Holy Land. The Knights Hospitallers of the Order of St. John of Jerusalem in the twelfth century C.E. offered aid to pilgrims and the sick throughout Europe, and at one time were active and held land in Rhodes, Cyprus, Italy, Germany, and England. If hospice workers were unkind to patients, or neglected them in any way, the workers were whipped and condemned to eat bread and water for a week.[1] The records of the Knights Hospitallers, which have been kept for six hundred years, show their efforts to maintain their ideals and goals, despite increasing wealth and land holdings. At their hospice, or hospital, in Rhodes, the incurably ill were sheltered and cared for apart from those with other illnesses, in a group of rooms reserved for travelers and pilgrims.

Since, in the medieval worldview, life and death were each considered part of the same mortal process, pilgrims and travelers were housed together with the dying. All were on a journey, and therefore needed a place to stop for comfort. The news that the travelers brought with them from the outside world was of value. The dying were also valued as individuals and as beings who were on the road to a higher plane of existence.

With the forced closure of monasteries in many countries during the Reformation, the concepts of hospice and hospital gradually became distinct. Today, the responsibility of caring for the sick and dying, formerly a private or religious one, has become a public or government function.[2] Although science has supported medi-

cine with marvelous discoveries to cure disease and prolong life, the modern hospital increasingly has the look
and feel of a laboratory. The bureaucracy needed to support the hospital system places increasing demands on
the time and energy of medical staff as well as patients.
The modern hospital, though well equipped to aid in an
acute, life-threatening situation, is seldom in a position
to offer comfort to a traveler who is nearing his or her
journey's end. Now, after a lapse of several centuries,
hospices are again caring for the dying and their families, due in large part to the work of Cicely Saunders in
London, England, and Elisabeth Kübler-Ross in the
United States. Dr. Saunders is the founder of the first
modern hospice in the world. She began her career as a
nurse and eventually became a physician. Queen Eliza-
beth II awarded Dr. Saunders the Order of the British
Empire for her work with hospice, thus elevating her to
the peerage and bestowing the title "Dame" (the equivalent of knighthood and the title "Sir" for a man).

In the late 1940s, Dr. Saunders became friends with
a man in his forties who was dying of cancer in a busy
London hospital. As they talked, the idea of a place that
could meet the needs of the dying, his needs, began to
grow. Together they shared the dream of a haven where
others like him could die in peace and dignity. This
man, who had escaped from the Warsaw ghetto, died in
1948. He bequeathed £500 to Dr. Saunders in order to
be, as he put it, "a window in your home."[3]

St. Christopher's Hospice (the name "hospice" had
been revived by the Irish Sisters of Charity, who began
opening homes for dying patients in the nineteenth century) grew from this gift, and from the work and plan-

ning of other donors over the next decade. St. Christopher's, which originally worked only with cancer patients, has continued to expand its services, including a Domiciliary Service Program, which offers in-home help for the family, and also educates staff, students, and visitors. It is from this model that other hospices have grown, both in England and in the United States. Financial needs are met partly by contracts with the National Health Service in England, with the remainder being made up by donations. True to the old hospice ideal, no patient is refused service because of inability to pay. "Giving care is St. Christopher's only way of fund raising."[4]

Patients with various terminal illnesses are admitted to the hospice at their doctor's request. Some come to stay, while others remain for a time, then return home. A few who have shown an improvement are sent back to a treatment hospital. Whatever the disease or the prognosis, all patients receive personal care and are greeted by name upon admission and throughout their stay. Bereaved families are supported by visits from St. Christopher's staff and volunteers. Relatives of deceased patients are remembered with anniversary cards the first year after bereavement, and are welcome to services at the chapel and to a monthly social club, as well as to general parties attended by staff and their families. Like residents of a small village, St. Christopher's staff, patients, and families share a feeling of community, a family feeling.

Dr. Saunders visited Yale University in the early 1960s to speak of her efforts on behalf of the terminally ill. With St. Christopher's now in full operation, a group of clergymen and medical people in New Haven, Connecticut, began efforts to develop an American hospice. Florence Wald, R.N., former dean of the Yale University School of Nursing, investigated the need for hospice in New Haven. Reverend Edward Dobihal, clinical professor of pastoral care at Yale New Haven Hospital, who had long been concerned about the care of the terminally ill in his ministry, also contributed to the study, which was completed in late 1969. The next few years saw incorporation, the formulation of a hospice philosophy, and a donation enabling hospice of New Haven to rent a small office and to hire Florence Wald and three others. Later, Dr. Sylvia Lack of St. Christopher's was hired as the first medical director.

Progress was slow, however. When local opposition prohibited land purchase for a facility, the founders realized that they needed to prepare and educate the public to receive hospice. Parents and families in Hamden, Connecticut, were concerned and afraid to have their children play near a place full of sick and dying people. These fears were unfounded, especially because the hospice was not slated to be an inpatient facility. No patients would be housed there; the location would merely serve as a central office which coordinated a home-care program. Approval came gradually. By mid-1974, patients were being served by the home-care program, and in autumn of the same year, funds were received from the National Cancer Institute and the Kaiser Foundation (a health maintenance organization in California). By late 1976, the community had given its full support.

The New Haven hospice was the first of three demonstration projects funded by the National Cancer Institute; the others were located in Boonton, New Jersey, and Tucson, Arizona. Two fundamental difficulties had to be faced: the American medical community's existing terminal care policy and the bureaucracy of contemporary health care. Planners feared that hospice ideals and goals would be compromised. Indeed, many in the medical establishment expressed doubts at first, thinking that hospice, and palliative home care particularly, would be unacceptable in this country. Planners were told that "when Americans are sick, they want to be in a hospital. Nobody dies at home in this country; the society isn't set up for it."[5]

But the response of patients and families has proved otherwise. A service emphasizing care rather than technology can be accepted by both lay people and professionals. Evaluation studies done between 1974 and 1976 show that hospice services measurably benefit patients and families. In a quasiexperimental control study that I conducted as a dissertation for the Yale School of Medicine and the National Cancer Institute I demonstrated that many people in this country do desire home care and are willing to make sacrifices and adjustments in order to keep a family member at home.

HOSPICE NOW

Since The Connecticut Hospice, Inc., New Haven, began serving patients in 1974, the concept has spread rapidly. Communities throughout the country have sought hospice services and are creating facilities. Based on information collected in the 1991 National

Health Provider Inventory, there are 951 hospices throughout the United States.[6] About a third of the hospices were located in six states: California, Illinois, Michigan, North Carolina, Ohio, and Texas. California had the greatest number of hospices (83), followed by Michigan (57), Illinois (49), North Carolina (48), Texas

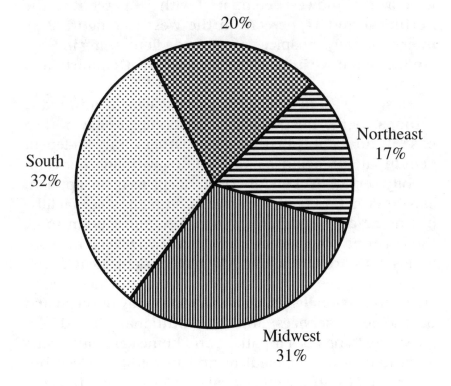

Figure 2.1. Percent Distribution of Hospices by Geographic Region.

Source: The data presented graphically here is from A. Jones, "Hospices and Homecare Health Care Statistics," *Advance Data* 257 (November 1994): 1–7.

(42), and Ohio (39). Florida, Minnesota, and New York each had more than thirty hospices. Fifteen states and the District of Columbia each had fewer than ten hospices. From the same study done in 1991, the majority of agencies were located in the South and Midwest regions; 39 percent were in the South and 29 percent were in the Midwest, compared with 18 percent in the Northeast and 14 percent in the West (see figure 2.1). Internationally, hospices are already flourishing in England, Germany, Cuba, Finland, Norway, Denmark, and Spain.[7]

Hospice is a flexible concept that can fit into many settings. Some hospices are functioning today with a base in an established hospital. Others have independent inpatient facilities or affiliations with another community service. Not all American hospices offer inpatient care at either a hospital or freestanding hospice facility, but home care and bereavement programs seem to be the norm. It would seem, then, that two divergent types of hospices are developing: (1) independent, heavily volunteer hospices with unstable funding in which a variety of professional staff deliver a wide array of social and psychological services; and (2) institutionally based hospices providing both inpatient and home care, supplying a greater variety of medical and nursing services but fewer social and psychological services. The latter employ a smaller number of volunteers and paid staff, and also experience fewer funding problems. A recent study done by the National Health Provider Inventory found that 5 percent of the 951 U.S. hospices were proprietary, 88 percent were nonprofit, and the type of ownership for 7 percent was government or other (see figure 2.2).

In 1986, Congress enacted legislation making hospice care an option under Medicaid, a federal program providing health care coverage to low income individuals and families, speeding access to hospice services. Currently thirty-six states have chosen to offer hospice benefit to Medicaid beneficiaries.[8] More and more hospices are becoming certified under Medicare (the health

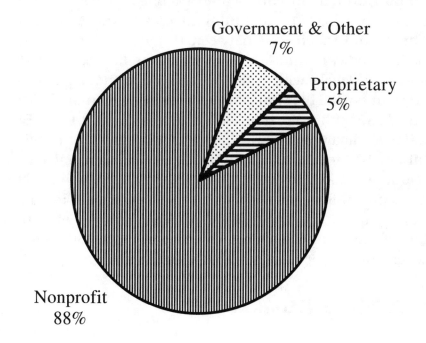

Figure 2.2. Percent Distribution of Hospices by Type of Ownership: United States, 1991.

Source: The data presented graphically here is found in A. Jones, "Hospices and Homecare Health Care Statistics," *Advance Data* 257 (November 1994): 1–7.

care provision of Social Security) and Medicaid; 67 percent of hospices were certified for Medicare and 57 percent were certified for Medicaid, and some are certified for both.

Current legislation may have a great affect on the growth of hospice. Republicans in the House of Representatives have pledged as part of their "Contract with America" that the federal budget be balanced by the year 2002. Entitlement caps would be used to restrain the growth of programs including Medicare and Medicaid. This would mean that between the years of 1996 and 2002, Medicare and Medicaid would be limited to 1995 spending levels with inflation and beneficiary number adjustments. This would mean drastic cuts in Medicare and Medicaid, cuts that would increase each year. By 2002 Medicaid alone would be cut 31.7 percent or $65 billion.[9] When considering budget cuts, special care should be taken to protect hospice, and to view hospice as a possibility for significant cost savings. Hospice home care is less expensive than institutional care any day of the week. On average a hospital costs $500 a day whereas hospice care costs only about $100 a day.

WHY DO WE NEED HOSPICE?

Although it is a cliché to say that today we live in a highly technological, bureaucratic society in which community and personal supports and traditions have broken down, nonetheless it's true. The needs of the dying and their families are personal, and those needs are not often met by the impersonal, highly specialized medical technology and the bureaucracy of the modern acute-care hospital.

Care should enable the terminally ill to continue as vital, functioning participants in life, and to maintain their identity and capacity to contribute as full human beings. Unfortunately, dying patients are often cared for in acute-care hospitals and institutional settings, where the structure, organization, and philosophy of the medical staff are geared toward aggressive cure. Practices in such facilities characteristically exclude the elements that are essential in the delivery of proper terminal care: involvement of the family in the patient's medical situation, which facilitates acceptance and alleviates potential guilt; care of the patient and family with respect to all relevant needs (physical, emotional, spiritual, and social); avoidance of heroic measures when such treatments are not warranted by the prognosis; effective use of narcotics for the alleviation of pain; execution of the patient's wishes with respect to environment and therapy options; and integration of the medical staff as a unified team into the process of maintaining the patient's total well being.

There is general accord among those examining current practices in the care of the terminally ill that existing institutional practice is usually deficient, inappropriate, limited, and in many cases devastating to the patient. David Shephard cites three reasons for the pervasive inadequacy of terminal care.[10] First, the emphasis on treatment and investigation leads the medical staff to regard the patient as a disease entity and not as a whole person. As Kübler-Ross has indicated, the patient "may cry for rest, peace, and dignity but he will get infusions, transfusions, a heart machine or tracheotomy, if necessary."[11] The patients are often inappropriately subjected to the rigors of curative therapy even when they are beyond the stage of possible recovery. At this time, whatever therapy is given should instead be geared solely to maximizing comfort.

A second factor in deficient terminal care is treatment in an inappropriate environment. In an acute-care hospital, the orientation of facilities, policies, and staff is toward cure rather than alleviating suffering, whereas hospice is by nature dedicated to meeting the everyday needs of its patients. Inadequate care may also be a consequence of the psychological inability of people in our society to confront the dying. Ironically, investigators have found that physicians are more fearful of death than members of any other occupation. Herman Feifel, one of the leaders in the field of thanatology and a professor at UCLA, is well published in the area of death and dying. He suggests that practicing curative medicine facilitates and reinforces the denial of death, thereby preventing physicians from comforting their patients and providing nonclinical, social, and personal support.[12]

The third factor underlying inadequate care in a health-care environment is the training of staff, which exacerbates rather than alleviates society's inability to confront or cope with death. Dehumanizing approaches to patient care result when staff anxieties intervene in the process of assisting the dying person. Defensive behavior by staff and friends, such as indifference, hostility, or detachment from the dying person, magnifies the loneliness of hospitalization and accentuates the withdrawal of the patient, who is already experiencing a diminished sense of self and a decreasing awareness of the environment. Interaction between patient and staff is strained further by the pressure of bureaucratic hospital procedures.

The tendency to quietly forget about patients once they are stigmatized with the label "incurable" can bring on a terrible sense of desolation. Patients may become overwhelmed with hopelessness, withdrawing into loneliness and depression.

Death in the acute-care setting represents a technological failure, not a natural and inevitable conclusion to life. Fortunately, due in part to the positive effects of Elisabeth Kübler-Ross's work, attitudes toward death have been reexamined and continue to be revised. With new attitudes may come a more humane and sensible approach to the care of the dying. To accomplish this completely, changes must be made in medical education. Many physicians believe that their routine care, aggressive treatment designed to cure a disease combined with a pleasant bedside manner, is the equivalent to hospice care. They do not understand the philosophy which dictates that both patient and family be considered the unit of care, and therefore integral to all aspects of the decision-making and treatment processes. Some doctors also tend to make the referral to hospice too late. When patients have only weeks or days to live, they cannot participate in treatment decisions or remain vital members of their households. These are outside the realm of possibility because time is too short. When a referral is made for patients who have fewer than six months to live, the hospice staff does not have enough time to work with them and treat them according to the hospice ideals. Unfortunately, although many enter medical professions for humanitarian reasons, doctors are often trained to cure their patients rather than to care for them. "What's happening in our medical schools and hospitals these days?" asks Dr. Morris Wessel, clinical professor of pediatrics at Yale University School of Medicine and a founding member of the New Haven Hospice. "You walk to the door, you leave your humanity outside. . . . Why did physicians stop paying attention to the human side of the patient? . . . The young doctors today need to understand that human beings die. It happens; that's reality."[13] *Caring is healing, no matter how long the patient lives.*

Hospices have an educational effect upon physicians. When the hospice is not housed in a hospital, there is a great opportunity to learn about palliative care, about the value of home visits and of interacting with dying patients. Physicians who continue to care for their patients after referral to an independent hospice are also learning these techniques. Naturally, other aspects of their practice are affected as well. With the comfort *and* cure of the patient in mind, physicians and nurses become willing to learn about symptom control from hospice.

Since the comfort of the patient is one of the prime reasons for the existence of hospice, it is also one of the reasons for hospice's popularity. Besides, many people prefer to die at home rather than in an institution. The patient's comfort does not rely exclusively on medications for pain or on corrective measures for distressing symptoms. It is also drawn from the environment: being comfortable, having familiar surroundings, loving care, and perhaps two kinds of visitors seldom seen in an acute-care setting—young children and pets. Comfort may also mean the freedom to live and die in the style of life that the patient has created.

The comfort of familiar surroundings, or a homelike inpatient hospice unit, benefits the family also. The patient in distress is not the only one suffering; the family suffers as well. One of the basic tenets of hospice care is the treatment of patient and family *together.* Death in acute-care institutions has caused many families to come apart; hospice helps to make death a coming-to-gether. Approaching death can be a spiritual and growth-filled experience for families. Hospice staff are trained to facilitate communication among family members so that the remaining time can be as complete as possible. Family problems cannot be ignored, for if they remain unresolved, they affect the peace of the dying person and the ability of survivors to help ease the dying process. When family members are able to express feelings, patients feel less isolated and freer to express their feelings as well.

Caring for the patient at home also affords survivors protection from the hazards of bereavement, which may include stress, depression, increased use of alcohol and other drugs, withdrawal, identity crisis, suicide, and loss of appetite. Research indicates that a significant difference exists in the mortality experience of grieving families, depending upon whether the patient died at home or in the hospital. The risk of a remaining relative dying within a year of bereavement was found to double if the first death occurred in a hospital rather than at home.[14]

For those cases in which the patient was cared for at home prior to death, the ability of family members to resist a devastating and prolonged period of grief can be attributed in part to the continued support of professionals who assisted in the care of the patient. Home-care situations also allow the family to witness the progression of the illness, making the reality of death easier to grasp.

The anticipatory grief experienced in a home care setting is also very valuable. Family members are able to begin mourning for the terminally ill patient before death has actually occurred. Although this may have negative aspects (at times the grieving person may ignore the patient and treat him as if he were already dead), anticipatory grief also allows the patient and family to mourn together and discuss their feelings. The blow is eased when death does take place. Home care allows those left behind to see that death need not be painful or lonely or agonizing. It can be beautiful, fulfilling, and a completion of a life well-lived.

The terminally ill person who is dying at home is still part of the whole community. This community of neighbors consists of varying ages and occupations, ranging from the postman to a visiting toddler. It is beneficial for relatives and children to witness the dying process at home and not be frightened by it. A positive experience at home can counteract the unnatural scenes of violent death that saturate the media. Many who have been present during a peaceful death fear their own mortality less.

After death has occurred, surviving family members receive continued care from hospice. Hospices in the United States and in England offer individual bereavement groups. This helps to prevent some of the loneliness that exacerbates grief. Mourners often experience isolation, and do not receive much understanding or tolerance from the rest of society. After the first flurry of activity following a death, the bereaved are likely to be left alone, and are expected to return to "normal" within a short time. We are beginning to recognize, however, along with changing attitudes toward death, that mourning is a necessary psychological process which can be aided by acknowledgment from the rest of the community. Hospices are invaluable in this process because the family is not abandoned after a member's death. The bereavement process cannot be avoided or curtailed, but it can be resolved by continuity of care.

We often think of the dying as "them" and the living as "us," as if we were separate. Among the moral and spiritual benefits of caring for a dying family member is the erasure of this distinction. We are all on the same journey, come from the same entrance, and leave by the same exit. We are all wayfarers on the road, and all of us need to stop for refreshment and comfort before the end of our journey. With hospice, we now have a choice about where we would like that stop to be.

NOTES

1. Sandol Stoddard, *The Hospice Movement* (New York: Stein & Day, 1978).
2. Ibid.
3. Herman Feifel, *New Meanings of Death* (New York: McGraw-Hill, 1977), pp. 159 and 161.

4. Ibid.

5. S. Lack and R. Buckingham, *First American Hospice: Three Years of Home Care* (New Haven, Conn.: Hospice, Inc., 1978), p. 4.

6. A. Jones, "Hospices and Homecare Agencies: Data from the 1991 National Health Provider Inventory (NHPI), Division of Health Care Statistics," *Advance Data* 257 (November 1994): 1–7.

7. Ibid.

8. National Association for Home Care, "NAHC 1995 Legislative Reports," *Blueprints for Action* (February 1995): 9–69.

9. Ibid.

10. David Shepard, "Terminal Care: Towards an Ideal," *Canadian Medical Association Journal* 115 (1976): 97–98.

11. Elisabeth Kübler-Ross, *On Death and Dying* (New York: Macmillan, 1969).

12. Herman Feifel, "Perception of Death," *Annals of the New York Academy of Science* 164 (1969): 669.

13. Stoddard, *The Hospice Movement.*

14. D. Rees and S. Lutkins, "Mortality of Bereavement," *British Medical Journal* (October 1967).

3

Contemporary Issues in Hospice Care

by Kate S. Mahoney*

The need for hospice will become more intense as we enter the twenty-first century. Modern technologies allow people to live longer, and the number of aging Americans is increasing as the Baby Boomer population ages. Here we examine hospice issues that need to be addressed as our society and its demographics change. All of the following issues have a unifying theme: *making hospice a choice for everyone.*

---

*Kate S. Mahoney is an associate field specialist for System Initiative in Math and Science Education. She holds a B.A. in Anthropology from the State University of New York at Geneseo and an M.A. in Curriculum and Instruction from New Mexico State University in Las Cruces, New Mexico.

MAKING HOSPICE AVAILABLE
TO ALL PEOPLE WHO NEED IT

Before taking a look at those people who need easier access to hospice, it's important to look at those who most commonly use hospice services. In 1992, a study showed that 53 percent of hospice patients in the U.S. were men, and 68 percent of them were sixty-five years of age or older. Of the women, 72 percent were over sixty-five.[1] It appears that both men and women equally participate in hospice, and the majority are senior citizens. Ethnically, the statistics show an imbalance among hospice patients. In a 1995 study, Lattanzi-Licht and Conner found that Caucasians constitute the vast majority of hospice admissions with 85 percent. Ethnically diverse groups make up the rest of the admissions with 9 percent of hospice patients of African American descent, 3 percent Hispanic, 1 percent Native American, and 2 percent all other racial groups. Upon examining these statistics, many questions surface about the exclusion of groups such as young adults, ethnically diverse cultures, and children. Why are these groups so underrepresented among hospice patients?

Child Social Security Beneficiaries

As shown above, hospice is most commonly used by white men and women over the age of sixty-five. Children are also victims of terminal illness such as cancer and leukemia, and these children need the long-term social, physical, emotional, psychological, and spiritual support that hospice has to offer. Unfortunately, a large number of children do not have access to Medicaid and therefore have little chance of affording hospice care. Almost 20 percent of the under-eighteen population has no private health insurance. Child Social Security beneficiaries are especially likely to be without health insurance because they are less likely than other children to have a parent with a job that offers health benefits. Child Social Security children, by definition, are the children of workers who are either retired, disabled, or deceased. The children are not eligible for Medicaid, and they are frequently deprived of even minimal health care.[2] An obvious solution is to make amendments to the Social Security Act to add children to the list of Social Security beneficiaries who can qualify for Medicaid.

Ethnicity

Statistics provided by the National Association for Homecare in 1995 showed that 85 percent of hospice patients were Caucasian. The other 15 percent consisted mostly of African Americans, Hispanics, and Native Americans, respectively. Clearly, these numbers are not proportional to current demographics in the United States. So why is it that cultures other than Caucasian only participate minimally in hospice?

We need to consider the different cultural values that exist among African Americans, Native Americans, Hispanics, and Caucasians. Each culture has its own definition of death, what it means to the family as well as the patient, and how dying people should be cared for. Hospice may offer services representative of traditional Caucasian dying values, which may not accommodate the needs of other cultures outside of this group. Another explanation may be that hospices are geographically located in areas more accessible to Caucasian people. Not many hospices are found in rural areas, on reservations, or in the inner city. Whatever the reason, it's important to be aware of who is using hospice and who isn't. Efforts need to be made so that hospice becomes an option for everyone.

Veterans

Under the benefits offered by the Veterans Administration (VA), terminally ill veterans don't have the same access to the full range of hospice services as other terminally ill Americans. In the past, veterans were authorized to receive home care, including the services of a home-care aide, at VA expense. The VA in 1983, under revised guidelines, discontinued authorization for home-care aide services, and several states since then have terminated services altogether or have limited them to a very small group of veterans.[3] Such financial restrictions have made it difficult for veterans to receive home care, but again, amendments can be made in legislation to require coverage of such services, including hospice, for all veterans.

Rural Areas

Although there are no statistics about city versus rural versus suburban, one area where hospice is not commonly found is in rural areas. The rural hospices which do exist may be outreach programs from an institution and sometimes they interface with visiting nurses' association or other home health agencies. Other rural hospices are strictly independent.

The cost and time that it takes to reach patients in rural areas make it very challenging for the hospice worker. It could take hours for hospice personnel to reach a patient and this becomes a problem when patients require two to three visits per day. Other obstacles that restrict hospice care in rural areas are the travel expenses, the time that it takes to reach rural areas, and road conditions. Some of the living conditions in remote areas could also inhibit the delivery of hospice services, especially if the particular area has no electricity and/or no access to water. Because of these obstacles, many rural patients are forced to use the inpatient hospital and nursing home facilities, options which pose their own special problems. The distance to the inpatient facilities can be especially hard on aged spouses, other family members, and on the hospice patient.

How can we reach people in rural areas more readily without losing the cost-effectiveness of hospice? One suggestion is to attract more facilities and personnel to these areas so that access to hospice is closer. A shortage of physicians and nurses exists. Rural America has 33 percent of the population, yet only 12 percent of the physicians and 18 percent of the nurses.[4] To attract personnel to rural areas, the government can offer loan forgiveness to student physicians and nurses or require an internship in a rural area as part of the medical and nursing school curriculum. Medicare could also serve as a solution if it offered reimbursement to compensate for the extra cost needed for hospice personnel to reach these rural areas.

REIMBURSEMENT

Though the loftiest goals of hospice soar to the heavens, it is rooted to the material plane; one does not exist without the other. Financial matters and reimbursement are necessarily of much concern. Hospice funding comes from a variety of sources: individuals and foundations, third-party payers (private carriers, Medicare, Medicaid, state and local government), and donations from groups such as United Way. As was mentioned earlier, the government recognizes the value of hospice both for humanitarian reasons and for practical ones. Hospice care for the terminally ill is less expensive than acute-care hospitals. Legislation makes it possible for hospice programs to receive reimbursement from Medicare and Medicaid. Yet many services are not covered by Medicare, Medicaid, or private insurance. Those services not covered include physician home visits, bereavement services, volunteer director services, homemaker services, intensive services, and education services.[5] Also, many insurance companies fund only aggressive treatment rather than extended palliative care. There are many terminally ill patients who are too young for Medicare and are not eligible for other programs.

In the United States, we have a tendency to fund institutional rather than home care, even though home care may be less expensive and more congenial. Currently, 85 percent of public funds are devoted to institutional care.[6] Medicaid, a state-run program, can fund home-care services for the elderly, but few states exercise that option. Although Congress is working on legislation to fund more home-care programs, institutional care still receives the greatest reimbursement.

The institutionally based hospice does not have the financial difficulties of the independent hospice, but usually does not offer as great a variety of social services. Financial considerations may compel many hospice programs to seek shelter within an institution and may affect other hospice decisions as well. Funding may require a particular staff composition—the use of registered nurses (R.N.s) rather than less expensive licensed practical nurses (L.P.N.s).

Currently, Medicare will not cover hospice visits where the reason for the visit is counseling of patients' families, even where the patients may be physically or mentally incapable of participating in counseling. The social and emotional problems of patients and their families are just as important as physical problems and need to be treated with equal concern and intensity. A social worker or informal caregiver's role is to resolve emotional and social problems, and these problems may be restricting the patients' treatment and recovery, so these services may save the institution money in the long run.

Another service that is important yet not reimbursed is

the expertise of a registered dietitian. As illness progresses, the terminally ill patient's nutritional needs will change, and decisions regarding force-feeding (intravenously) or even withholding nutritional support must be made. The advice of a dietitian is essential at such times. Also, over 50 percent of the elderly living independently in their homes have nutritional deficiencies, and the services of a dietitian could help prevent and treat many diseases including diabetes, osteoporosis, and high blood pressure.[7] Inclusion of these benefits may prevent a home care patient from seeking a more costly institutional setting.

RECRUITMENT OF HOSPICE PERSONNEL

With the demand for hospice increasing, there is a need to encourage appropriate use of therapists and hospice personnel. In institutional settings, one in six physical and occupational therapy and one in eleven speech pathology positions are now vacant.[8] Because of this, hospice will be competing with other home health agencies and institutions for staff. Federal and state regulations should be passed to promote the use of nurse practitioners, physician attendants, and other qualified home health personnel in home care.

As mentioned before, another way for hospice to increase the number of qualified staff is to require medical students to have a hospice internship as part of their graduate medical education. Medicare pays for the training of medical residents and interns at virtually all hospitals in the United States. We need the same application to hospice care.

STAFF STRESS

Staff "burnout" can be a hazard for anyone in the "helping" professions and for health-care workers particularly. Burnout could cause withdrawal from patients, which is especially detrimental to hospice work. Team coordinators are aware of this and many of the programs that are basic for hospice work offset the staff stresses which can lead to burnout. In many ways, hospice is a less stressful environment than others in which death occurs. For example, there is no conflict between prolonging life and allowing death to occur, a frequent source of staff stress in an acute-care setting. Also, everyone on the staff is committed to hospice philosophy, which sees death as a natural occurrence and the comfort and peace of mind of the patient as the highest priorities. Staff assignments allow enough time to facilitate this peace and comfort and to allow for expressions of caring that are satisfying to patient and staff: for example, when staff takes the time to sit and talk and listen. Positive relationships with patients, families, and other staff members, as well as positive community support and approval compensate for the intensity of the work and ensure staff satisfaction. Flexible scheduling which allows for time off and work rotation also helps.

The team structure has many built-in safeguards against burnout. The thorough orientation everyone receives inculcates a clear expectation of what the work will involve. In-service education, including workshops, seminars, and lectures about the fundamentals and philosophical practice of hospice care keeps the skills of health care professionals, M.D.s, R.N.s, and lay volunteers updated and can fill any needs for information the staff may have. Case management meetings allow for the contribution of each team member and also serve as a hospice review, ensuring that the program is meeting its goals for each patient and family. Staff support meetings offer guidance to hospice workers on how to deal with a number of both clinical and nonclinical issues. Topics such as problems that staff may be having with a family, another agency, hospitals, or doctors are discussed and plans of action are determined. Staff support meetings strengthen the interaction of team members. The patient and family need support and so does the staff.

SYMPTOM CONTROL

Hospice strives to maintain dignity while providing palliative care for the terminally ill patient. A recurring issue, therefore, is the need for continuous education in symptom control among the staff. Stressing the importance of symptom control is necessary most importantly for the patient's comfort but also for a commitment to the hospice philosophy. Symptom control does not apply only to pain; it includes many other things as well. Good skin care through the use of water mattresses, sheepskin pads, rubs, and frequent changes of position, can prevent or clear up bedsores. Good mouth care prevents sores and infections. Bowel function is also important to the bed-bound patient. Constipation, a frequent side effect of many analgesics, may be helped by prescriptions (included with the pain medications), enema, and removal of fecal impaction. There are many distressing symptoms that the team needs to be aware of and know how to treat: urinary problems, nausea and vomiting, shortness of breath, coughing and the possibility of choking, sleep difficulty, diarrhea, edema (swelling), ascites (fluid collecting in the abdominal cavity), and itching, to name a few. Even though a cure is no longer possible, there is still much the medical team can do. The team needs to be educated and skilled in symptom control, as well as the application of hospice philosophy on a daily basis.

PAIN CONTROL

Much chronic pain is perpetuated by "PRN" prescriptions used by physicians. The letters stand for the Latin phrase *pro re nata* meaning "whenever necessary," and dictate that the patient be given medication at the onset of pain. The problem lies precisely here, for medication should instead be given prior to the onset of pain. When severe pain is experienced and expected to continue indefinitely, patients enter a world of horror and hopelessness that for those treated by conventional means ends only with death. When medication is not administered until the onset of pain, patients must experience pain while waiting for medication, and they continue to experience it while waiting for the medication to take effect. Then the process begins again when the next onset is experienced. Dying patients already feel enough loss without having more of their independence and limited time sacrificed because the pain has returned.

Since pain control is so important to its philosophy, the hospice staff have become knowledgeable about the management of pain. Even so, more education is always needed in this area in order to continue to improve the comfort of patients and their families. Increased and expanded education in the area of pain management will also allow the staff to continue to update its methods with respect to this extremely important component of the hospice philosophy.

AWARENESS TO PERCEPTIONS OF GOOD CARE

It is vital to discuss the perceptions of patients, families, and staff members regarding the qualities needed by a caregiver in order for hospice to be effective. The need for a caring and compassionate staff is essential to patients, their families, and the bereaved. Patients also need to have care tailored to the individual, particularly regarding pain and symptom control and physical care. Because hospice centers on the idea of teamwork, the preconceptions and priorities of each member of the team must be discussed, understood, and then integrated to provide a program of care that will most benefit the terminally ill patient.

There is another quality, not mentioned by the groups surveyed, which I believe to be important: humility. We "caregivers" can become egotistical and overvalue our own importance. We forget how privileged we are to be able to serve and how much our patients give. As all of us know, egotism closes the heart and prevents real communication. Those who are close to death, and their families, teach and give so much, and we can receive their lessons best when our hearts are open. Those of us who work in a hospice situation are truly fortunate, for we have many opportunities to learn life's deeper lessons.

EDUCATION OF THE MEDICAL STAFF

Physicians need to continue education in home health care and especially in the area of pain control. Two of the many topics which need to be addressed include improving the comfort of the terminally ill patient and the discovery of new, less intrusive medical procedures. Current pain control methods need to be improved for the benefit of patients and their families, if the commitment of hospice to its primary philosophy is to be maintained. This education needs to focus not only on technical advances in medicine, but also on philosophical or attitudinal advances. Communities reluctant to accept a hospice locally and doctors who are unwilling to refer patients to hospice care need to learn what hospice programs truly entail and how such programs only benefit communities and patients.

More research needs to be undertaken to improve hospice care services. Incentives should be given to promote such research, and professional conferences need to be held regularly in order to exchange findings. Workshops, symposiums, publishing more health care journals, and offering incentives for medical students to chose hospice care as a career are all ways of offering education to our physicians. Physicians will play a vital role in the continuing growth of hospice as a professional health care system.

HOSPICE CARE FOR PERSONS WITH AIDS

Most hospice programs don't offer care for people with AIDS, although, with the epidemic our country faces, we need hospice to incorporate care for these patients. Why is it, then, that these services are not available to persons diagnosed with AIDS?

One reason for the lack of AIDS care in hospice could be that with the demands already on hospice from other terminal illnesses such as cancer, the personnel and facilities needed to provide hospice services just aren't available nor are the funds to support new services. The message here is clear: because you have AIDS, there is not enough room for you.

Perhaps it is a subconscious way of discriminating against persons with AIDS. Health-care professionals may have difficulty treating AIDS patients because AIDS has been considered by many to be a "dirty disease" contracted by homosexuals and intravenous drug users; for some, the pariahs in our society. Many people believe that persons with AIDS have brought the infection on themselves and therefore they do not deserve compassion. Others tend to classify AIDS cases as either "innocent" victims (such as infants, hemophiliacs, and other transfusion recipients) or "guilty" victims (including IV-drug users and homosexuals).[9] It is difficult for health-care workers to escape society's prejudices. Large sectors of society still condemn homosexuality and fail to come to terms with the nature of addiction. Because many of the addicted turn to crime to support their habits, addiction becomes synonymous with criminality in the eyes of many.

The need to address the AIDS epidemic remains acute. Education about AIDS, although a controversial issue, reaches our high schools, middle schools, and even some elementary schools every day, yet the number of people with AIDS is growing steadily. It is an issue here and now, for everybody, with or without AIDS, homosexual or heterosexual. Hospice is designed to assist terminally ill people, and AIDS patients qualify for the same consideration that is given to other terminally ill people.

LACK OF BROADER HOSPICE ORGANIZATION

Despite the amount of time which has elapsed since the concept was introduced, hospice in the United States still occurs as a local phenomenon. Although individual hospices may be well-organized, what is necessary is a private state association of hospice programs. Each state would have its own hospice which would provide a key location for hospice agencies to come together.

Each state is culturally different and therefore has different needs. The needs of people along the border of Mexico are different from the needs of people in inner-city Boston. Urban and rural issues would be taken into consideration in these state agencies, as well as different cultural values and attitudes regarding death.

A state agency could more quickly address the situation of a crisis. For example, the Hanta virus that caused nearly eighty deaths in New Mexico in the early 1990s is a situation where a state hospice could have taken action. The bereavement services by hospice could have been provided to the survivors, and also to those involved in the Oklahoma City bombing disaster in April 1995. By having a state association of hospice programs able to react quickly and appropriately to these issues, the victims and families of victims can receive improved care in a timely and organized manner. Goals of a state association would include unifying states to form an alliance for support. This could be a place for hospice workers to come together and share experiences, hold conferences, exchange ideas, and discuss political issues facing that particular state.

DELIVERY OF BEREAVEMENT SERVICES

After death has occurred, surviving family members receive special care and attention from the hospice team. Hospices offer individual bereavement support, including follow-up visits by staff members and bereavement groups. Currently hospice provides friendly visits at ninety days after death and at 180 days. This varies among hospice programs, where some provide only one friendly visit after the death of a loved one. Much more needs to be done to determine the number of friendly visits to be made to families who have experienced the death of a loved one.

Not enough research is yet available on the bereavement process itself. Mourners often experience isolation, and do not receive much understanding or tolerance from the rest of society. After the first flurry of activity following a death, the bereaved are likely to be left alone, and are expected to return to "normal" within a short time. Many effects of these feelings are increased use of alcohol and barbiturates, possibly leading to addiction. By becoming more sensitive to the needs of the bereaved, many health problems and addictions can be avoided. The efforts of the entire hospice team can help survivors make the transition from the death of a loved one back into their own, fulfilling lives, but more information on grief and mourning is necessary in order for bereavement programs to provide the best possible services.

NOTES

1. Lattanzi-Licht and S. Conner, "Care of the Dying: The Hospice Approach," in *Dying: Facing the Facts,* eds. H. Wass and R. Neimeyer (Washington, D.C.: Taylor & Francis, 1995), pp. 143–62.

2. National Association for Home Care, "NAHC 1995 Legislative Reports," *Blueprints for Action* (February 1995): 9–69.

3. Ibid.

4. Ibid.

5. R. Buckingham and D. Lupu, "A Comparative Study of Hospice Services in the United States," *American Journal of Public Health* 72 (1982): 455.

6. National Association for Home Care, "NAHC 1995 Legislative Reports."

7. National Association for Home Care, "NAHC 1995 Legislative Reports."

8. Ibid.

9. G. Friedland, "Clinical Care in the AIDS Epidemic," *Daedalus* 118 (1989): 67–78.

4

Hospice Administration

Everyone on the hospice staff, including physicians, nurses, and other medical personnel, receives training. All staff members are given help in exploring their own feelings about death and loss, as well as discussing feelings about working with the terminally ill and about palliative care rather than cure.

All of the team (including patients and families) need to understand and accept the concept of palliative care as the major medical goal; the inappropriateness of resuscitation attempts and life prolonging techniques; and the acceptance of death. These are all fundamental to the basic philosophy of everyone on the hospice team.

Figure 4.1 illustrates the structure of a typical hospice organization. This chart shows how policy filters down

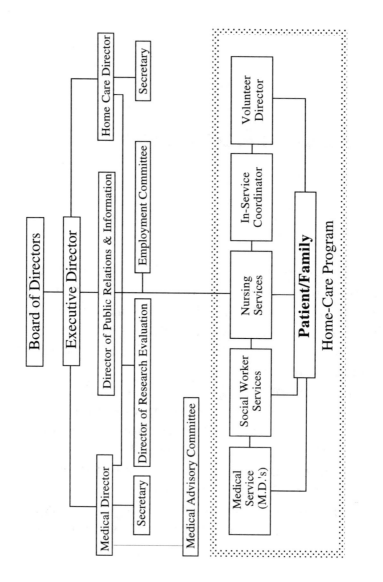

Figure 4.1. A Typical Hospice Organization Chart.

Source: R. Buckingham, *The Complete Hospice Guide* (New York: Harper & Row, 1983).

from the board of directors through the executive director and various committees to the patient and family.

ADMINISTRATION

The administration within a hospice, especially the executive director, is an important part of the effectiveness of the multidisciplinary team, with the administrator serving as a liaison with the board of directors, the medical director, and the director of the home-care program. The executive director recommends policies for the hospice to the board of directors, but the board has final say on all policies, from hiring and employment standards to community relations. The administrator represents hospice when working with other health-care agencies and when speaking to members of the community. The administrator understands and has a commitment to hospice care and its patients and families. Combining the fundamental caring attitudes of hospice with necessary practicalities, the administrator needs to have skills in public relations and developing funding resources.

MEDICAL DIRECTOR

The medical director is a liaison between the hospice and the medical community. The personal physician continues to plan his patient's medical care, but may consult the medical director regarding symptom control. The medical director may refer the patient to other facilities when appropriate (such as radiation therapy for pain control, or an acute-care setting if needed). The medical director is coordinator of the multidisciplinary team and must have a thorough understanding of the needs of the terminally ill. He has a commitment to hospice philosophies of care, and shares this with other members of the team.

NURSING STAFF

The nursing staff is supervised by the medical and home care directors and is headed up by a director of nursing. The director is responsible for instructing the staff as to the hospice's nursing policies and practices and selecting patients and families to be matched with individual nurses.

Nurses need medical skills for symptom control, pain relief, and more, for each nurse is a teacher as well. They are assigned to a patient and family to train the primary care person within that family in tending the patient. This requires considerable skill, for the nurse (particularly in home care) may direct or assist in the patient's care, but also encourages the primary care person to perform that care directly. Nurses are in close contact with the patient and family, and in the home-care setting they may be the most frequently seen member of the team. Helping with the patient's care, visiting the family, and weathering the crises of terminal care together bring nurse and family close. The nurse is given many opportunities to assess the patient's and family's needs and to communicate with them. The high level of interaction, plus the high level of nursing and communications skills required in terminal care, necessitate a high nurse-patient ratio. It is desirable that there be one nurse for each for patient and family unit.

It may be that the best hospice nurse is a licensed practical nurse (L.P.N.) rather that a registered nurse (R.N.). Today's R.N.s are highly trained scientifically, and are sometimes reluctant to perform the more menial tasks necessary to keep a terminally ill patient comfortable. Preferring to use only those skills within an R.N.'s training (giving medication, for instance) can keep an R.N. from being a flexible hospice nurse. L.P.N.s also have a wide range of skills and are generally willing to do whatever the situation demands. This adaptability makes the L.P.N.s very useful amid the changing events of terminal care. Needless to say, there are many R.N.s who are wonderful hospice nurses, but it would be advisable to have a large proportion of L.P.N.s on the staff as well. Reimbursement systems may make this difficult, however, as some sources will only pay for the services of an R.N. Restrictive third-party reimbursement may dictate staffing.

DIRECTOR OF VOLUNTEERS

In addition to the medical director and the director of nurses, hospices need a director of volunteers, because volunteers play an exceedingly important role in hospice work. As I have previously discussed, volunteers must be screened in private interviews, trained, placed, and supported. Hospices usually do not receive reimbursement for volunteer services, yet volunteers enable hospice to offer a richer variety of programming than would otherwise be possible. The multidisciplinary team needs all its members.

STAFF STRESS

As was mentioned earlier, staff stress and "burnout" are issues which need to be addressed in all of the "helping professions," but particularly in hospice care. The emotional drain of working with terminally ill patients must be addressed by team coordinators, as the withdrawal that results from stress is especially detrimental to hospice patients.

The hospice philosophy, which views death as an integral part of life, is espoused by all the team members. Positive relationships with patients, families, other staff members, and the community help compensate for the intensity of the work. Staff scheduling that ensures time off and regular work rotation reduces burnout. In-service programs, including lectures and seminars designed to teach coping strategies, as well as staff support meetings, also strengthen the team members and ease tension.

5

Cost of Hospice Care

THE EMOTIONAL COST

Hospice care acknowledges the extraordinary cost of commitment to this meaningful service to others. That is, it acknowledges the emotional, social, and psychological costs that burden patients and their families. Often these costs, many of which can continue long after the death of the patient, weigh heaviest on the survivors. To date, they have not been adequately measured.

When a loved one dies, for example, there will be those left behind who increase their use of medications and/or alcohol to escape the pain of their loss. Sometimes a family member will continue this effort to numb the pain until an addictive pattern arises. The cost in

83

emotional well-being is difficult to measure, and it may be more expensive than all the dollar costs of physical care. The costs could begin to mount as workdays are lost and personal or family income suffers. If this weren't enough, there are the hidden costs of family disruption following a death, and an increased divorce rate among parents who have lost a child.

Inherent in hospice are many costs and benefits that go beyond funding sources and the expense of care. These relate to both patients and families. When they are treated in a hospital, patients give up much of their right of self-determination. Hospitals are institutions in which patients are categorized according to their condition and treatment is determined by the immediate prognosis. Since hospitals are not designed to care for dying patients, such an environment tends to exacerbate the feelings of "contamination" that terminally ill patients often experience. Nursing procedures may also contribute to these feelings. Standard attention to sanitary practices may be incorrectly interpreted by patients as being directly related to their medical condition. Because medical intervention is limited for the terminally ill, physician visits are often short and may appear to result in little tangible benefit for the dying patient. Physicians tend to delegate more time to other, nonterminal patients, for whom medical intervention has some visible and gratifying result.

As for the families, visits with a patient in a hospital are often not as casual as they should be. Family members aren't quite sure what to say, and patients aren't comfortable revealing their emotions so each assumes standardized roles of behavior. Meaningful personal exchange is further handicapped by interruptions from the hospital staff and consideration for other patients. A frequent problem for treatment of the terminally ill in hospitals is the often haphazard assignment of "roommates." What kinds of psychological implications arise in terminally ill patients when their roommates recover from one or another acute condition? The doctors pay more visits and spend more time with patients who are on the mend. Also, the hospital staff tends to give more attention to those who are recovering, in part out of reluctance to face death and the dying process. Can staff members handle the frequent question: "How much longer must I go through this?" Since most people in a hospital are not there with a terminal illness, the hospital staff may not be experienced in handling what many health professionals see as a "defeatist" concept of dying or the acceptance of death.

Hospice care, on the other hand, deals directly with the concerns of the dying, addressing the special considerations of terminal care. In addition, there are special functions performed by hospice staff which are often overlooked in an acute setting. Treated in a home hospice environment, patients are part of the total household. They are able to witness and often to participate in real-life events such as meal-making, family discussions, and other daily routines. This provides a vital link with life. Seeing that life is a continuous, ongoing process provides some comfort to those facing death. Also, the home provides a setting more congenial to intimacy with family members and hospice staff.

Several issues must be considered before home hospice care is selected as the course of treatment. One is the loss of wages by family members who take time off from work to care for their loved one. Are there financial alternatives or ways to augment the family income? Furthermore, involvement in treating the dying can be emotionally draining and is often exceedingly traumatic. Family members may also face ethical decisions regarding care given to the dying person. For example, should oxygen be given in the final stages of the disease when breathing becomes irregular and shallow, or should "nature" be allowed to take its course? Then again, should efforts at pain control be intensified even if by doing so, the patient's death is hastened? Finally, the moment of death and its aftermath may be traumatic. The body of a loved one turning dark from lack of oxygen may recur in the mind of the survivors long after the patient has died.

Once these situations are addressed by the caregivers and acceptable solutions found, home hospice care provides valuable spiritual and psychological benefits. Witnessing the natural death of a loved one enables us more easily to handle our own inevitable mortality. Death is not to be feared and avoided but rather embraced as the final moments of a life process. Also, special insights and intimate thoughts are often shared in the relationship between dying persons and those they leave behind. From a psychological standpoint, those families who participate in home hospice care don't usually experience the feelings of guilt that relatives sometimes report after the death has occurred. The family members as caregivers are comforted in the knowledge that they were directly involved in attending to their loved one in that person's time of greatest need.

The presence of family members during the patient's final moments of life afford a peaceful and tranquil end accompanied by people who genuinely care. At this time, family members are together in an environment in which they can immediately express their thoughts and feelings with one another, which in turn sets up a framework for mutual support during the bereavement process.

COST OF HOSPICE CARE

Hospice is increasingly seen as an attractive alternative to the high-tech, high-cost, cure-oriented care for patients with terminal illnesses. Much research has been done to determine whether or not hospice is cost-effective care. Although most research shows a savings for patients using hospice, other studies show no significant difference in cost effectiveness.

The results of a study of the effect of the hospice program on Medicare Part A expenditures during the first three years of the program reported that Medicare saved $1.26 for every dollar spent on hospice care. That is, for every $2.26 spent by Medicaid on traditional methods of care, only $1 was spent to provide hospice care.[1]

According to Bischoff, Medicare reimbursement for hospice increased in 1990 and was expected to continue for the next five years, which shows that hospice is increasingly viewed as a more feasible alternative to hospital care for many.[2] Interestingly enough, the longer the length of stay for a patient, the more of the costs Medicare will pay. Medicare reimbursement for patients enrolled in hospice for less than thirty days did not always pay for their care, although Medicare reimbursement for patients enrolled in hospice for greater than thirty days usually exceeded the costs of care resulting in a small profit for the hospices.

In a 1993 study done by Bischoff, a model allocating costs for fifteen service components was developed using data from fifty-two patients receiving Medicare hospice benefits in a home-care environment. Medicare patients were chosen for this study because, when segregated by payer, they comprise the majority of hospice patients in this population.[3] The service components consisted of visits by the administrative nurse, registered nurse, chaplain, counselor, home health aid, social worker, volunteer coordinator, physician office visits, durable medical equipment, outpatient services, pharmaceuticals, medical supplies, and miscellaneous expenses (e.g., ambulance). Bischoff found that reimbursement for hospice care in 1990 was $75.80 per day for up to 365 days of care; much less than cost of hospital care per day.

Overall, most studies have shown positive results of hospice care on the experience of dying patients. Perhaps any variations in findings reflect differences in the quality of hospice care offered throughout different regions of the United States.

COST OF HOSPICE FOR PERSONS WITH AIDS

In 1995, the Centers for Disease Control and Prevention reported that AIDS is the leading cause of death of

American men between the ages of twenty-five and forty-four, and the third leading cause of death for American women in the same age group. The disease ranks fifth among causes of death of children under the age of fifteen. By 1994, 1,052,000 cases of AIDS had been reported to the World Health Organization (WHO). In February 1995, WHO estimated the actual number to be closer to 4 million, 2.5 million of which are located in sub-Saharan Africa. By the year 2000 WHO expects there will be 30–40 million cases of AIDS worldwide. Approximately 13 million people are infected with HIV, the virus which causes AIDS (although symptoms of the disease itself may not yet be evident), and an estimated 6,000 new people become infected every day.[4] The current and future cost of care for persons with AIDS (PWAs) and HIV infection continues to be of great concern.

AIDS affects primarily young adults in their twenties, thirties, and forties. The number of cases is increasing among intravenous (IV) drug abusers, minorities, and infants.[5] Increasing numbers of homeless PWAs have been noted, particularly among those who are IV-drug abusers. With no cure or even a viable vaccine in sight, most individuals die within two years of being diagnosed with AIDS. Treatment for persons with AIDS has typically occurred in acute hospital settings. This is very costly, and places a strain on the capacity of hospitals in the areas most heavily affected.[6]

Increasingly it has been recognized that AIDS patients could be treated in alternative settings. Individuals suffering the terminal stages of AIDS could benefit from hospice services. Hospice, with its emphasis on palliative and supportive care, is an appropriate and cost-effective alternative to the much more expensive and much less empathic acute hospital setting. There are a variety of settings where hospice care can be provided to meet each individual PWA's needs.

GENERAL COSTS FOR PWAs

Over the past few years, researchers have attempted to estimate the medical costs of persons with AIDS. These estimates have varied considerably depending on the definition of AIDS used, the scope and definition of costs, and the time period and geographic area studied.[7] The initial report on the cost of treating PWAs by the Public Health Service's Centers for Disease Control in 1985 forecasted a cost of $147,000 per AIDS patient from initial diagnosis until death. This estimate was based on 168 inpatient days and an average survival time of about thirteen months.[8] Subsequent studies reflect much lower lifetime medical care costs and reduced hospital stays. In 1988, estimates of the lifetime medical care costs per PWA from diagnosis to death ranged from between $55,000 and $80,000.[9] Compare this to an estimate made in 1994 by the National Association for Home Care: the lifetime cost of treating an AIDS patient was approximately $102,000. In this way, the cumulative cost of treating all persons with HIV will increase 48 percent from 1992 to 1995, rising from $10.3 billion to $15.2 billion.

These estimates, however, do not provide a complete picture of the cost of care for persons with AIDS. Many studies have excluded nonhospital costs such as drugs, ambulatory and ancillary services, long-term care, hospice and home health care, counseling, and other community services. There are limited data available on the use and costs of medical care for IV-drug abusers, women, and pediatric patients. In addition, much less is known about the costs incurred by HIV-infected individuals who have not yet developed AIDS. As a result of these shortcomings, the cost estimates to date most likely underestimate the full economic impact of AIDS.

The Cost of AIDS: Some Preliminary Considerations

The total costs associated with AIDS including both direct and indirect costs were estimated to have reached $66.5 billion in 1991, of which $56 billion, or approximately 84 percent, represents indirect costs.[10] Indirect costs reflect the losses incurred as a result of the disability or premature death of working-age adults. These costs could rise even higher in the future: transmission of the virus has not yet peaked, and the percentage of HIV-infected individuals who will develop AIDS continues to increase.[11]

The medical management of AIDS care has changed and will continue to change over time, although whether this will lower or raise medical care costs presently remains unclear. There are reports that AIDS patients are less likely now to be admitted to intensive care units than they were previously and that the average length of hospital stay has declined.[12] A reduction in hospital use has been attributed to alternative modes of health care delivery which rely on outpatient care and community-based services. The cost of these services will need to be evaluated in order to analyze the implications of relying less on hospitalizations and more on community support services.[13]

The introduction of new treatment approaches will also influence costs. One such example is the widespread use of zidovudine (AZT). AZT has been found to decrease the incidence of life-threatening pneumonia in persons with AIDS, which may ultimately reduce medical costs by eliminating or shortening lengths of hospitalization. Alternatively, AZT may increase treatment costs. It is an expensive drug (costing between $8,000 and $10,000 per patient per year) and requires close medical monitoring. As many as 30 percent of AIDS patients on AZT may develop severe anemia and require regular blood transfusions. Although AZT appears to increase the life expectancy of AIDS sufferers, they may still die from other AIDS-related disorders, such as dementia, which can be even more expensive.[14]

Because complications resulting from AIDS appear to differ among high-risk groups, changes in the number and patterns of people contracting the disease could influence the cost involved.[15] Early in the epidemic, the majority of AIDS cases were homosexual or bisexual males; but now the trend is changing, with an increasing proportion of IV-drug abusers, women, minorities, and children being noted.[16] These changes in the demographic profile of people with AIDS will have a dramatic effect on health resources and medical costs in certain metropolitan areas. For example, more than 75 percent of the nation's pediatric AIDS cases have also occurred in these cities.[17] The costs associated with caring for people with AIDS who are IV-drug abusers and children with AIDS are considered to be higher and more likely to be social rather than medical.[18] Oftentimes these patients remain in an acute-care setting longer because they have no one to care for them or they do not have a suitable place to go when they are discharged.

Changes in the geographic distribution of the AIDS population may also have an impact on the costs of care. What sort of impacts, however, is difficult to predict. In the early stages of the epidemic, New York and San Francisco accounted for 34 percent of U.S. AIDS cases, but as the epidemic has continued to spread, this has diminished to 20 percent. Clearly there has been a shift to smaller urban centers that may not have health care delivery systems adequately equipped to provide the care most people with AIDS need.[19] Additionally, it has been found that hospital costs are lower in the West than the Northeast, and that these variations are caused partly by differences in the average length of hospital stay (twenty-four days in the Northeast versus fourteen days in the West). Differences in patient diagnosis appear to explain most of the variation in length of hospitalization. The incidence of IV-drug abusers with AIDS is higher in the Northeast, thus accounting for longer lengths of stay and more days per year than in the West.[20]

Finally, along with the uncertainties about overall costs per se, there are growing concerns regarding the source of funding for care. Recent studies demonstrate a shift from private to public financing, with 40 percent of all people with AIDS, and up to 90 percent of all children with AIDS, being served under the Medicaid program. In states like New York and New Jersey, the proportion may be as high at 65 percent to 70 percent.[21] The estimated cost of providing AZT alone will exceed $120 million.[22] Even so, there are concerns that Medicaid coverage is inadequate to meet the needs of most individuals. States have flexibility in determining which services they will reimburse; this may mean that some states are meeting the needs of persons with AIDS more effectively than others.[23] Concern has also been voiced about the impact this will have on state finances and on the Medicaid program in general.[24] As more money is allocated for AIDS care, Medicaid coverage for other groups could be restricted.

The increasing number of AIDS cases and the cost associated with new treatments will undoubtedly place a tremendous burden on the health care delivery system as it currently exists. To date, medical management of the illness has been primarily in the inpatient setting. This is not only costly, but often medically necessary. Many times AIDS patients remain in acute settings when there is no medical need because of the lack of appropriate alternatives.[25] In order to reduce the cost of care for persons with AIDS, effective alternatives to hospitalization, such as hospice or visiting nurse associations and other home health agencies that practice the philosophical concepts of hospice care, will need to be utilized.

The progression of the AIDS illness varies for each patient. Some individuals die soon after diagnosis. For others, the illness is chronic with periods of acute illness, interspersed with long periods of relative stability during which time they may be able to work. Most persons with AIDS will require inpatient hospital services at some point during the course of their illness. The rest of the time they can be maintained at home with home-care services. Other people with AIDS, particularly those suffering from AIDS dementia complex, may require institutional care.* People with AIDS in the terminal stage of the illness could benefit from hospice services.

Many communities are developing comprehensive care systems similar to San Francisco's approach, which combines acute hospital AIDS treatment units with community services. This system is considered to be the most effective approach to providing care to the person with AIDS over the course of the illness. San Francisco utilizes a continuum-of-care model, which includes a designated hospital AIDS unit, a hospital-based outpatient clinic, and a comprehensive network of home and community-based services.[26] Lifetime medical care costs for AIDS patients in San Francisco have been lower than in other areas of the country as a result of fewer hospitalizations and shorter lengths of stay.[27] This experience has been widely attributed to the effective use of community-based services such as home care, hospice, and support services. Additionally, San Francisco utilizes a network of trained volunteers who assist patients with meal preparation, light housework, transportation to clinic appointments, or provide relief to caregivers.

---

*AIDS dementia complex is chronic mental deterioration which impairs social and occupational functioning. Many AIDS patients suffering from this condition experience memory and abstract thinking loss.

Three major concerns must be addressed before hospice will gain wider acceptance as an alternative to current treatment by people with AIDS and their families, hospice providers, and the public: (1) defining and determining a market for hospice, (2) demonstrating cost effectiveness of hospice care compared to current alternatives, and (3) assuring third-party reimbursement for hospice care.

HOSPICE AS AN ALTERNATIVE: SOME WORKING MODELS

Over the past decade, the use of hospice services has moved into the mainstream of cancer care. Legislation passed by Congress in 1982 provided for ongoing federal reimbursement for hospice and was predicated on the assumption that hospice care for dying patients resulted in lower health care costs.[28] Since 1982, Medicaid and other third-party payers such as Blue Cross/ Blue Shield and various health maintenance organizations have also been providing reimbursement for hospice services.

AIDS is similar to cancer and other terminal illnesses in that hospitalizations are most frequent in the early and late stages of the illness. Thus, as with other terminally ill patients, reduced costs for persons with AIDS can be achieved by providing more relevant palliative care in lieu of hospital services during the final months of life. The hospice service package includes: pain and symptom control, pastoral or spiritual counseling, bereavement services for patients and their families, twenty-four-hour, on-call nurse and counselor, and respite for caregivers. These services have been effective for other terminally ill patients, and are equally suitable for people with AIDS and their families. Hospice teams can utilize their present knowledge related to symptom management, death and dying, and bereavement needs of family and friends to expand their programs for the terminally ill person with AIDS.

As noted above, hospice services have been utilized by AIDS patients in San Francisco as an alternative to hospitalization since the early stages of the epidemic. Evidence of this is the expansion of Shanti, a hospice organization that, prior to the AIDS epidemic, gave help and emotional support to terminally ill patients, and that now provides its services almost exclusively to people with AIDS.[29] It appears that the demand for these services is growing. In 1986, the AIDS Home Care and Hospice Program in San Francisco increased its daily caseload from eighteen patients initially to sixty-three patients in 1986, with a waiting list of thirty to forty-five patients.[30] With the growing number of AIDS patients, the caseload will continue to increase into the twenty-first century. Over 90 percent of AIDS cases served by this program have died at home, while 10 percent have died in a hospital or have been discharged from the program when hospice services were no longer needed.

San Francisco's experience demonstrates that a market for home hospice services for persons with AIDS exists and is best suited for individuals who have a supportive network of friends and family available to assist with their care. Some terminally ill patients, however, cannot be maintained at home because they do not have friends or family available to assist with their care, or because they do not have a place to live. In such situations the patient requires residential care or housing. Hospice programs are now developing creative approaches to meet the needs of these individuals by providing their services to people with AIDS who are living in group homes, or in some instances developing their own residential hospice facility to meet the needs of terminally ill AIDS patients in their community.

Residential hospice facilities that are often associated with existing hospice home care programs are also being utilized to care for the terminally ill person with AIDS. These facilities were designed to provide a greater intensity of services with a home-like atmosphere for the patient. They are suitable for the terminally ill who can no longer be maintained at home because of inadequate support systems, or for individuals who require a significant amount of skilled nursing or attendant care. They provide an ideal setting for the person with AIDS exhibiting cognitive impairments, ranging from short-term memory loss to full dementia in advanced stages which requires twenty-four-hour supervision. These residential facilities are reimbursed at the Medicare/Medicaid established inpatient hospice rate, or through negotiated rates with third-party payers. This rate is higher than the routine home-care rate, but much less than that of acute hospitalization.

The group home residence model and the inpatient residential facility are two examples of the way hospice programs have adapted their services to meet the needs of the AIDS patient. However, the extent to which hospice programs will be able further to expand their services will depend on acceptance of the hospice philosophy by people with AIDS and their families. Some AIDS patients may not be ready to accept palliative care only, and may choose to seek aggressive therapy for each opportunistic infection.* With AIDS affecting primarily a younger population, the introduction of new therapies provides hope for survival despite the predicted short life expectancies. Therefore, hospice programs that can be flexible and allow the use of experimental drugs or provide services to individuals living alone will be more attractive to people with AIDS.

THE COST OF HOSPICE CARE VERSUS HOSPITALIZATION

The next area of concern for hospice care is that of demonstrating its cost effectiveness compared to standard available alternatives. Very few studies have analyzed the cost effectiveness of services enabling AIDS patients to remain at home and out of institutions for as long as possible.[31] Only one study to date has evaluated the cost effectiveness of a home-based hospice program for people with AIDS. Although the results were positive, the study looked at patients residing in one geographic area only. It needs to be determined whether or not these results can be duplicated elsewhere.

---

*Opportunistic infections are caused by organisms that are normally present in humans, but do not cause disease unless the immune system is damaged. An opportunistic infection occurs after the microorganism or virus, normally held in check by a functioning immune system, gets the chance to multiply and invade host tissue.

Research studies on the cost effectiveness of hospice care for terminally ill cancer patients have generally been encouraging. Savings have resulted from substituting less costly home care for acute care during the final months of life.[32] One striking example of such savings appeared in a study comparing the costs of the last two weeks of life for patients dying in the hospital versus those dying at home. The study found hospital costs to be 10.5 times greater than home-care costs. The higher cost was found to be attributable to the greater use of diagnostic and therapeutic services.[33]

A 1988 study by Mor and Kidder found similar results. They compared the costs of both hospice home care and hospital-based hospice programs to those of conventional care for terminal cancer patients. The greatest savings were noted in the last month of life. The cost of treatment for conventional care patients was nearly three times as high as that of home-care hospice patients. Overall costs for the last year of life were lower for home-care and hospital-based hospice patients than for their conventional care counterparts. Again, the difference in costs was attributed to the substitution of home-care services for inpatient care and a reduction in the intensity of ancillary service use for hospital-based hospice patients.

A San Francisco study evaluating the effectiveness of a home-based hospice program for people with AIDS found it to be far less expensive than inpatient hospitalization.[34] The study found that the 165 AIDS patients who received hospice care from this program during fiscal year 1985 required an average of forty-seven hospice days per person at an average per diem cost per patient of $94, for a total cost per patients of $4,401. Although this was not a randomized, controlled study, the implications for cost savings are great when compared to the costs to AIDS patients of treatment at San Francisco General Hospital. There the average per diem cost was $773; the average cost per hospitalization, $9,024; and the total lifetime cost for patients who received all their care at San Francisco General Hospital, $27,571.[35] Additional data from San Francisco estimate the cost of available alternatives to home-based hospice for people with AIDS to be much higher. Chen's study, as cited in Landers and Seage, estimated the average cost of acute inpatient care at $800 a day; sub-acute care at $500 a day; a skilled nursing facility at $300 a day; and a residential hospice at $100 a day. These comparisons further demonstrate the magnitude of the cost-effectiveness of home-based hospice programs.

Alternatives to acute hospitalization for AIDS patients include any of the following: home care, home-based hospice care, hospice care provided in a group home or inpatient residential facility, or institutional care in either chronic hospitals or skilled nursing facilities. Any of these settings are appropriate and needed in order to prevent people with AIDS from being hospitalized in acute-care settings. The most appropriate setting for AIDS patients will depend on their care needs, home environment social support network, insurance coverage, and community setting.[36] Because of the nature of the illness, any one of these settings may be appropriate for a person with AIDS at any given time.

For individuals who require twenty-four-hour care and who cannot be maintained at home, placement in a hospice inpatient residential facility or an institutional setting becomes necessary, although the availability and cost of such options will depend on the community where the patient resides. The following estimates were made by Benjamin in 1988: (1) the cost of a chronic care hospital is $500 a day; (2) an inpatient residential hospice facility, $350 a day; and (3) care in a skilled nursing facility can range from $125 to $200 a day.* Still, all these options are far less expensive than an acute-care facility, where costs can range from $800 to $1,000 a day.[37] When asked, most people with AIDS would prefer to remain at home or in noninstitutional settings rather than in hospitals or nursing homes. While the lower cost of a nursing home may make it appear to be a more desirable alternative, experience to date has demonstrated a reluctance by both AIDS patients and nursing homes to accept this option. People with AIDS prefer to be in a homelike environment with individuals who are closer to their own age. There are a number of reasons why nursing homes have not been used. The current high occupancy rate in nursing homes enables administrators to select the patients they wish to admit. Many nursing homes do not have the staffing capacity, and they are concerned about the additional cost of providing the physical and psychosocial care AIDS patients require. Current nursing home rates are already considered to be inadequate by the industry.[38]

Home-based hospice services can be utilized by the AIDS patient who prefers to remain at home. Most pro-

---

*More recent information is not easily accessed, but it stands to reason that although the actual numbers may now be higher, the savings realized through hospice care will be proportional.

grams provide services to those who live alone as long as they have someone who can be available to help if needed. This alternative is not only cost-effective but also provides such services as attendant care; volunteer support; bereavement counseling; and twenty-four-hour, on-call nurse coverage. These services are all critically needed to maintain the patient at home.

Hospice services will not be acceptable to all AIDS patients. Even when homebound, some patients will continue to seek treatment aimed at cure. These patients can receive home-care services offered by a visiting nurse association. Both programs provide similar services and are often combined within a single agency. However, there is an important distinction between these two types of services. Home-care services are aimed at treatment of acute problems with the individual patient considered the unit of care. Insurers will reimburse skilled care only, and as such will not reimburse for social work services or bereavement counseling. Hospice services encompass both the physical and emotional needs of the individual and are provided to the entire family.

CASE STUDY

"Michael," a twenty-seven-year-old married man with two children ages two and five, was admitted to a hospice program after discharge from the hospital. Michael was diagnosed with AIDS and mycobacterium avium intracellular (MAI)* approximately one year previously,

---

*MAI is an opportunistic bacterial infection common to AIDS patients that can involve the gastrointestinal tract, lungs, bone marrow, or liver.

and prior to admission had been maintained at home with the support of home-care services. Since his diagnosis, he had received intermittent skilled nursing visits to monitor medication compliance, nutritional status, and blood work.

Michael was hospitalized for treatment of pneumocystis carinii pneumonia (PCP), malnutrition, and anemia secondary to use of AZT. Despite treatment, his physical status continued to deteriorate. Recognizing that treatment was no longer working, Michael requested to be discharged so that the could be at home with his wife and children. He had been hospitalized for fifty-four days, with total charges amounting to sixty thousand dollars, or approximately eleven hundred dollars a day.

A nurse and social worker from the hospice program made the first home visit together. The nurse assessed Michael's physical care needs and arranged for daily home health aide services to assist with bathing and ambulation. The social worker discussed Michael's concerns with him. Michael had not been able to pay his rent and had just received an eviction notice; his wife had not been able to work because she had no one to assist with child care.

The social worker spoke with the landlord and arranged to have the family stay in the apartment for one more month. The hospice program paid the rent for that month with donations, while the social worker continued to look for housing. The social worker consulted with the AIDS coordinator at the local AIDS service organization, who found subsidized housing for the family. The hospice program provided family counseling and child care through volunteers. Michael's status steadily improved; after two months he was discharged from the program as services were no longer needed. Michael has been receiving biweekly nursing visits for administration of medications. He is no longer homebound and has remained out of the hospital for the past six months.

This case study highlights several important points about the appropriateness of hospice care for AIDS patients. First, it demonstrates the commitment of a hospice program to assess the needs of the individual and to provide resolutions when possible. In this case, the hospice program was well integrated into the community and was able to access volunteers and resources from other agencies. Second, it demonstrates the unpredictable course of the AIDS illness. Michael was considered to be in the terminal stages of the disease; however, his prognosis improved quite dramatically without curative treatment. Whether or not this can be attributed to hospice services is unclear. But, the hospice program was able to remove the significant stress factors from Michael's life. As a result, Michael was able to concentrate all his energies on himself, further evidencing that when people are permitted to make their own autonomous choices about death, some actually live longer. When placed in a supportive atmosphere, many "terminal" patients improve significantly—their will to live improves dramatically. Third, the cost-effectiveness of hospice services for this individual were significant. The cost of home-based hospice care is less than $100 a day, which is less costly by far than care in an inpatient or chronic care facility. Additionally, Michael has remained out of an acute-care facility for six months. Finally, this case study demonstrates the useful application of two different home-care services. Hospice, with its integrated network of resources and services aimed at palliative care, was more suitable than home-care services during the terminal stages. Home-care services were effective when Michael required only skilled care.

Another major concern to be discussed in hospice care for people with AIDS is third-party reimbursement. Private insurers concerned about the high costs of medical care for AIDS patients are increasingly willing to reimburse for optional services that can be demonstrated to be both cost-effective and appropriate alternatives to hospitalization for their clients. Hospice care is an optional benefit, therefore, which most insurance policies cover. Typically, insurance companies deal with clients on an individual basis, and they review alternative treatment plans submitted by hospital discharge planners or social workers in community agencies. The insurer will reimburse the alternative service requested if it can be demonstrated to be cost-effective. The following is an alternative treatment plan developed by a hospital discharge planner and submitted to the patient's insurance company.

CASE STUDY

"John" is a thirty-six-year-old man in the terminal stages of AIDS hospitalized in an acute-care facility. Over the course of his hospitalization John has received treatment for PCP, cytomegalovirus (CMV)*, oral thrush, malnutrition, and dehydration. John has made the decision to cease curative care, and he is now ready for discharge pending approval of appropriate placement. John requires long-term placement for twenty-four-hour attendant care and administration of intravenous DHPG (ganciclovir) to prevent blindness secondary to CMV. John is confined to bed. He has frequent episodes of explosive diarrhea. He is too weak to feed or bathe himself. Because of John's care needs, he cannot be maintained at home. Discharge would normally be to a chronic-care facility where his acute-care needs can be met. However, John has requested to be transferred to an inpatient residence hospice facility in his community.

The sole purpose of this alternative treatment plan is to cover the cost of the patient's admission to an inpatient hospice facility that is approved by Medicare and licensed by the state. The daily cost will be $380 inclusive of most medications. This fee includes twenty-four-hour skilled nursing care, room and board, and any durable medical equipment the patient may require. Based on a seven-day week, the estimated cost will be $2,660 a week or $10,640 a month. John will also receive intravenous DHPG three times a week at an estimated cost of $70 per dose. Estimated costs will be $210 a week or $840 a month. The combined estimated monthly cost will then amount to $11,480.

Total charges to date at the acute-care facility are $67,979, based on forty-six hospital days, or $1,478 a

---

*CMV is a virus related to the herpes family. CMV infections may involve the eyes, lungs, central nervous system, and gastrointestinal tract. The disease can be treated, but it cannot be cured.

day. It is anticipated that the patient would have been routinely admitted to a chronic-care facility at an estimated cost of $567 a day, $4,250 a week, and $17,000 a month. The alternative treatment plan requests transfer to an inpatient residential hospice facility, which reflects an estimated cost savings of $1,380 a week or $4,520 a month. After review of the alternative treatment plan, the insurance company approved transfer to the inpatient residential hospice.

This case demonstrates the high cost of hospital care for persons with AIDS during the terminal stages of the illness. It is not uncommon for people with AIDS to continue to seek aggressive treatment aimed at cure for as long as possible. Additionally, some AIDS patients may need to remain in very costly acute-care facilities because of the lack of appropriate alternatives. This case also demonstrates the willingness of third-party payers to negotiate rates with hospice providers, thereby ensuring adequate reimbursement. This patient's care needs are such that he could not be maintained at home. If home hospice care was an appropriate alternative, the cost savings would have been much greater. The cost of home hospice care is less than $100 a day, which is dramatically lower than the cost of chronic care.

Finally, there is anecdotal evidence that Medicare and Medicaid's reimbursement rates may not be adequate to cover the cost of care for the AIDS patient. These rates were designed to cover the cost of caring for the terminally ill cancer patient. The cost of providing care for people with AIDS is often high as a result of increased costs for medications and attendant care. The cost of medications for cancer patients averages $10 to $15 a day, while the costs of medications for people with AIDS averages $45 a day. It is estimated that the average yearly cost of treating a person with AIDS is $38,300 and the average annual cost of treating a person without AIDS is set at $10,000.[39] Hospice providers are reimbursed by Medicare and Medicaid at a per diem all-inclusive rate, and as such are unable to bill separately for medications or equipment. If John had been a Medicaid recipient, the hospice program would have had to absorb the $210 weekly cost of providing DHPG to the patient. Frequently the person with AIDS, because of neurologic impairments, requires between eight and twenty-four hours per day of attendant care. Based on current reimbursement rates, hospice programs can only provide up to twenty hours of attendant care per client per week. Hospice programs often substitute volunteer care when possible. However, if the AIDS patient requires skilled care, they will provide the additional coverage and absorb the extra cost.

The high costs of caring for people with AIDS within Medicare and Medicaid's present reimbursement structure could place a strain on hospice providers. Medicaid currently covers the cost of care for 40 percent of all people with AIDS, and up to 90 percent of all children with AIDS. Eligibility for this program is limited to those with severe disabilities and income limitations. This coverage includes mandatory home care and optional hospice services. The Medicaid program pays almost 25 percent of the aggregate cost of all national expenditures for medical care on behalf of these individuals. The combined federal and state Medicaid expenditures for AIDS-related care in

1993 were estimated at \$2.5 billion. These outlays are projected to reach \$3.8 billion per year by 1997.[40]

Medicare coverage is even more limited and amounts to less that 2 percent of the total national cost of direct medical care for persons living with AIDS, an estimated \$385 million in 1993. Persons with AIDS must qualify for this program by first qualifying for Social Security Disability and Insurance and then waiting twenty-four months after his or her SSDI payments begin. Medicare services also include other home care as well. Medicare's share of treatment costs is expected to rise as new medical technologies and drugs enable persons living with AIDS and HIV-related conditions to survive the twenty-four month waiting period.

Many individuals with AIDS, however, have no private health insurance because they become unemployed or are not eligible for Medicare or Medicaid. Needed health care services are thus extremely difficult, if not impossible, to obtain. Many hospitals, home-care agencies, and other health care providers provide uncompensated care, but relief is desperately needed.[41]

SUMMARY

Hospice, with its emphasis on coordinated care, including intensive home-care, counseling, and support services, is one viable option along a continuum of care which should be offered to AIDS patients. Support for these services appears to be increasing among people with AIDS. Many, however, are not ready to accept the terminal status of the illness. Although there is no cure to date, the introduction of new treatments has prompted many persons with AIDS to continue to seek aggressive medical treatment.

The costs associated with medical care for people with AIDS are high. Concern over the increasing numbers of AIDS patients who will require services and the subsequent strain this could place on the current health system has prompted expansion of alternative settings to acute and chronic hospital care. Hospice has been demonstrated to be an appropriate and cost-effective alternative to hospital care for these patients. With its broad service package, hospice care can be provided in many different settings to meet the needs of the person with AIDS. Many hospice providers have already developed innovative programs for people with AIDS.

Hospice care demonstrates, through both tangible and intangible costs and benefits, its viability as an alternative to the chronic-care institutionalization of the terminally ill. However, for hospice care to be a widely used resource, its proponents must deal with society's negative feelings toward death, dying, and AIDS.

NOTES

1. H. Birnbaum and D. Kidder, "What Does Hospice Cost?" *American Journal of Public Health* 74 (1992): 689–97.
2. W. Bischoff, "A Cost Allocation Model for Hospice," *Nursing Management* 24, no. 12 (1993): 38–41.
3. Ibid.
4. World Health Organization, *Bridging the Gaps:*

1995 World Health Report (Geneva: World Health Organization, 1995).

5. J. Johnson, *AIDS: An Overview of Issues* (CRS Report No. 1B87150) (Washington, D.C.: The Library of Congress, 1991).

6. M. Merlis, *Acquired Immune Deficiency Syndrome (AIDS): Health Care Financing and Services* (CRS Report No. 1B87219) (Washington, D.C.: The Library of Congress, 1990).

7. J. Sisk, "The Cost of AIDS: A Review of the Estimates," *Health Affairs* 6, no. 2 (1987).

8. A. M. Hardy et al., "The Economic Impact of the First 10,000 Cases of Acquired Immunodeficiency Syndrome in the United States," *Journal of the American Medical Association* 255, no. 2 (1986): 19–31.

9. Institute of Medicine, "Care of Persons Infected with HIV," in *Confronting AIDS: Update 1988* (Washington, D.C.: National Academy Press, 1988), pp. 93–121.

10. A. Scitovsky and D. Rice, "Estimates of the Direct and Indirect Costs of Acquired Immunodeficiency Syndrome in the United States, 1985, 1986, and 1991," *Public Health Reports* 102, no. 1 (1987): 5–17 and 3102–3106.

11. Sisk, "The Cost of AIDS."

12. G. Seage et al., "Effect of Changing Patterns of Care and Duration of Survival on the Cost of Treating the Acquired Immunodeficiency Syndrome (AIDS)," *American Journal of Public Health* 80, no. 7 (1990): 835–39.

13. Sisk, "The Cost of AIDS."

14. A. Scitovsky, "Studying the Cost of HIV-Related Illnesses: Reflections of a Moving Target," *Millbank Quarterly* 67, no. 2 (1989): 318–46.

15. Sisk, "The Cost of AIDS."

16. Scitovsky, "Studying the Cost of HIV-Related Illnesses."

17. P. Arno, "The Non-Profit Sector's Response to the AIDS Epidemic: Community-Based Services in San Francisco," *American Journal of Public Health* 76, no. 11 (1986):1325–30.

18. Scitovsky, "Studying the Cost of HIV-Related Illnesses."

19. J. Green et al., "Projecting the Impact of AIDS on Hospitals," *Health Affairs* 6, no. 3 (1987): 19–31.

20. D. Andrulis et al., "The Provision and Financing of Medical Care for AIDS Patients in the U.S. Public and Private Teaching Hospitals," *Journal of the American Medical Association* 258, no. 10 (1987): 1343–46.

21. Institute of Medicine, "Care of Persons Infected with HIV."

22. W. Roper and W. Winkenwerder, "Making Fair Decisions about Financing Care for Persons with AIDS," *Public Health Reports* 103, no. 3 (n.d.): 305–308.

23. Merlis, *AIDS: Health Care Financing and Services.*

24. Sisk, "The Cost of AIDS."

25. L. Beresford, "Alternative Outpatient Settings of Care for People with AIDS," *Quarterly Review Bulletin* 1 (1989): 9–16.

26. P. Kawata and J. Andriote, "NAN—A National Voice for Community-Based Services for Persons with AIDS," *Public Health Reports* 103, no. 3 (1988): 299–304.

27. A. Scitovsky, M. Kline, and P. Lee, "Medical Care Costs of Patients with AIDS in San Francisco," *Journal*

of the American Medical Association 256, no. 22 (1986): 3103–3106.

28. V. Mor and D. Kidder, "Cost Savings in Hospice: Final Results of the National Hospice Study," *Health Services Research* 20, no. 4 (1988): 407–22.

29. E. Howell, "The Role of Community-Based Organizations in Responding to the AIDS Epidemic: Examples from the HRSA Service Demonstration," *Journal of Public Health Policy* 12, no. 2 (1991): 165–73.

30. J. Martin, "Ensuring Quality Hospice Care for the Person with AIDS," *Quality Review Bulletin* 10 (1986): 353–58.

31. S. Landers and G. Seage, "Medical Care of AIDS in New England: Costs and Implications," in *The AIDS Epidemic: Private Rights and Public Interest,* ed. P. O'Malley (Boston: Beacon Press, 1989), pp. 257–72.

32. A. Benjamin, "Long-Term Care and AIDS: Perspectives from Experience with the Elderly," *Millbank Quarterly* 66, no. 3 (1988): 415–43.

33. B. Bloom and P. Kissick, "Home and Hospital Cost of Terminal Illness," *Medical Care* 18, no. 5 (n.d.): 560–64.

34. Arno, "The Non-Profit Sector's Response."

35. Scitovsky, Kline, and Lee, "Medical Care Costs."

36. Beresford, "Alternative Outpatient Settings."

37. Benjamin, "Long-Term Care and AIDS."

38. Beresford, "Alternative Outpatient Settings."

39. National Association for Home Care, "NAHC 1995 Legislative Reports," *Blueprints for Action* (February 1995): 9–69.

40. Ibid.

41. Ibid.

6

Hospice Care for Children

THE NEED FOR HOME CARE

From the inception of modern medical care, hospitals have been the setting for the treatment of children with a terminal illness. The benefit of any continued hospital care is increasingly questioned once it is understood that there is no chance of the illness becoming controlled. The trend today is toward alternative care, and in the case of the terminally ill child the trend is home care. More and more advantages are being found in relation to the quality of care that the child receives and the psychological benefits for the family.

In the past, hospitals have been the appropriate place for the ill to be cured and the terminally ill to die. There is no question that the hospital is where the best possible medical treatment can be received. No other institution has the power to prolong life or resuscitate the dying individual. People, however, are increasingly rejecting hospital care in favor of being allowed to die with dignity and in comfort. Probably one of the most ignored segments of the terminally ill population, insofar as having this desire fulfilled, is the youth of our society.

The hospital, though known for its power to care for the sick, has never been strong on giving the psychological support the patient needs. In the case of the dying child, the hospital seems to promote anxiety and discourage its relief. Terminally ill children react more strongly than might be expected to changes in their environment, such as fighting between the parents, changes in school, moving, or separation. The hospital, then, would seem the last place to put the dying child for comfort and prolonged care. The most affected children, emotionally, are those of grade-school age who do not believe that a hospital is for their own well-being. Instead, they feel they are being punished for the prospect of their own death; their parents are sending them away to die.

Once hospitalized, the pressures of separation and loneliness continue to mount for children. They may be subjected to either partial or total isolation, making it even more difficult for them to adapt to their situation.[1] This feeling is further reinforced when, in the hospital, continuous care and regular visits by a doctor rarely occur. Instead, care is provided by several physicians and there is no continuity. Children then have no one they can identify as their physician, and the patient-physician relationship, which can be so important, is never established.

Home care for the dying child avoids much of the emotional stress of the hospital. This was especially evident when children dying of cancer "who were old enough to express an opinion, all preferred being at home to being in the hospital."[2] By being at home, children receive a variety of both psychological and social benefits. They are in a family environment where activities that have always been a part of their lives are taking place. The attention and discipline that they are accustomed to is not withdrawn as may occur in the hospital, and this can avoid confusion and unhappiness. At home, children receive the needed security and love that are intrinsic to the close family environment.

In the hospital, the affection that children need is often not provided. Terminally ill children want and often require more affection. However, they do not always make this need known. Instead of perceiving this greater need for affection, the parents of these children perceive quite the opposite. When this need for love goes unnoticed, children become lonely and frustrated.[3] This is less likely to occur in the home, where there is no nurse who must see to the needs of a number of other patients, or a doctor who has other appointments to keep. At home, families can share responsibilities for the care of a dying child, as well as provide love and affection. So, just as the home is the natural place for children to be while living, it can also be a natural one for dying: children have their parents with them, they are in an environment of family surroundings, they can eat foods they are used to, they are able to pursue normal activities as much as possible, and they can have the company of their brothers and sisters. By providing a more relaxed atmosphere, hospice and home care settings make terminally ill children more at ease and self-assured. This, in turn, helps children confront death more sensibly and enables them to spend the time they have left (which may be increased because anxiety has been reduced) more productively.

HOSPICE CARE FOR THE DYING CHILD

The benefits of most hospice programs are limited to adults, and approximately 70 percent of these adults are over sixty-five years of age.[4] But what about children with terminal illnesses? Do they not also need the special comprehensive and individual care that a hospice organization has to offer? Admittedly, the needs of children and their families are different from and more varied than those of adults, and integrating child care into a regular hospice program could be quite difficult. However, it seems that children, too, and their families, should have the possibility of receiving adequate and intensive total terminal care, which can rarely be found in today's massive hospitals.

Potential difficulties in providing hospice care for children could be that there are very few people specialized in hospice care for children. There may also be a reluctance on the parents' part to enter hospice for this would mean the beginning of the end for their child.

The term "child" covers such a wide range of stages in emotional, psychological, social, and intellectual development that it is difficult to speak about the child as opposed to the adult. However, to generalize, one could state that a child has not yet reached the levels of emotional, psychological, and intellectual maturity that are expected in most normal adults. Children's actual levels of development between the ages of birth and eighteen years will vary much more drastically than adults' levels between the ages of eighteen and ninety. Thus, children are less in control of their own situation in the world (the amount of control increasing with age) and are, to varying degrees, dependent on a parent or other adult figure (the degree of dependence decreasing with age). For the most part children are much more egocentric than adults, demanding and needing much more individual attention. Children have not learned to control the world around them as adults have, nor have they learned to conceptualize and objectify themselves and their situation. Children perceive everything that happens in their world to be a direct result of their own actions. Therefore, they cannot understand why bad things happen to them and those they love. Again, these factors vary drastically with age and state of development. One must keep in mind that growth, change, and development are the very essence of childhood, and it is for this reason that it is much more complex than adulthood. Although the distinctions pointed out above between child and adult are simplistic indeed, even these play a significant role in determining the different relationships a child and an adult will have with impending death and the different methods of care needed to deal with each.

In the past, children were practically never actively involved in their own treatment. The last few years have shown a tremendous change in understanding the attitudes of dying children and have consequently altered the whole approach to the terminally ill child. The most significant changes originated in Switzerland approximately thirty years ago, with the revelation that children's spontaneous drawings reveal much of their inner knowledge and awareness of ill health and preconscious awareness of impending death. The children internally realize that they may die, and although they have not verbalized their knowledge, it is expressed in their drawings. Dr. Elisabeth Kübler-Ross has used this method of spontaneous drawings with dying children over the last twenty years, and it can be used by any counselor, trained therapist, or physician in order to become more aware of children's inner knowledge of their terminal illness, as well as of their prognosis. This knowledge, which can be obtained within ten minutes, has changed the entire approach to the dying child. We can now communicate with children in symbolic verbal and nonverbal language, which makes it possible for children to reveal their inner knowledge to the adults around them. The therapist or counselor acts as a catalyst between parent and child.

In most cases, when all medical means have been used and all medical-scientific resources have been depleted, the children ask to be allowed to go home. For example, children share verbally or nonverbally, in plain English or in symbolic language, whether they are willing to continue chemotherapy. This is not just a reaction to the discomfort of treatment; it is also a result of their inner knowledge that further treatment will not produce additional benefits. Children and parents should meet with the therapist, who understands the symbolic language of the child, to discuss the child's discharge from the hospital for either home or inpatient hospice care.

It seems self-evident that terminally ill children need and would benefit from hospice care as much as, if not more than, terminally ill adults. Children's and their families' needs differ from those of adults in several respects, and a comprehensive program like that of a hospice could help fulfill those specific needs. First, children are not expected to take part (again depending on age and maturity) in the decision-making process of their own care. It is usually the family that takes the responsibility of decision-making, although the consequences will affect the child; thus a hospice's customary practice regarding the patient and the family as a single unit of care would be especially beneficial in caring for the dying child. Since terminal illness in children is less frequent and seems more "unjust" than terminal illness in adults, families of young patients have even more difficulties in dealing with and accepting the situation. As Dr. Morris Green states, "There are few human experiences so shattering as a child's death."[5] Therefore, the family would need trained emotional and psychological advice during, and most important, *after* the course of terminal illness. Another important point about children is that their reactions to their own impending death understandably vary greatly. The difference between the reactions and needs of two children of different ages or even the same age can be as great as that between child and adult. For example, some children may focus on the dying process (whether it will be painful, its duration, etc.) while others may center more on what will happen after death, both to them and to those they leave behind. These concerns will vary based on age and on the children's grasp of the concept of death, and also among children of the same age, based on upbringing (children raised in a religious home may focus on the idea of an afterlife, for example) and the children's own personalities. Therefore, an effective care program would require staff trained to deal with children not only on the medical level, but on psychological and emotional levels also, because most children (depending on age and maturity) usually cannot be directly confronted with the fact of their death. It is even more important that their daily lives retain as many aspects of their previous normal lives as possible. This, too, may put a greater burden on the parents, who may often feel the need to pretend that everything is all right with their child. Since the child is so reliant (depending on age) on the family and because of the need for a semblance of normality, it seems that, whenever possible, terminal care should take place in the home. Something like the hospice home-care programs, with the addition of specially trained staff to meet the psychological and emotional needs of children of all ages, would appear to be the ideal answer to children's terminal care.

It is only in exceptional circumstances that home care is not sufficient at the end of a child's life. Inpatient hospice units can better serve those families who may have inadequate environments for home care; e.g., those with small, crowded quarters; those with many small children who also need care; those without an adult who could care for the dying child; or families with battered children. These relatively rare cases will require a hospice inpatient unit. These units are small facilities that do not require separate buildings or administrations, which would make them economically unfeasible. Instead, they are affiliated with existing hospitals or clinics whose equipment and space they utilize for the time it takes to serve the needs of the end-stage period of the terminally ill child.

The palliative care unit of the Royal Victoria Hospital in Montreal is an example of an administrative compromise between the framework of a children's hospital and an independent hospice. These special palliative care units, or miniature hospice units, for children must have a totally independent staff with special awareness of the needs of the children. There must be rooms for parents, siblings of all ages, and grandparents, so that they can visit at any time of day or night. Ideally, these units should have adequate kitchen facilities where the family could prepare special meals, if necessary, for the dying child. There should be sleeping facilities with some privacy for the family, especially when the child is close to death. Adequate playrooms are also necessary, not only for visiting siblings, but for the interaction between siblings and the terminally ill child. Additional facilities for supplying music are also important, especially for a terminally ill adolescent. Enough resource persons are needed, not only for the physical care of these children, but for their emotional, spiritual, and intellectual needs as well. These units could be run at economically reasonable rates and would not only benefit families with insufficient home-care facilities, but would give families who are caring for their child at home a much-needed rest for a few weeks. This would allow parents to recuperate from home care and get a break when the terminal illness is of long duration.

The crucial and inherent bond between child and parent and the deep anxiety evoked in an adult by the dying child are two major factors that indicate the dire necessity to incorporate care for the family into the care given to the child. As Dr. Green points out, the dying child often awakens one of our deepest fears—death before fulfillment.[6] The experience of a child's terminal illness probably causes more psychological problems in families whose members are aware of the situation without being able to share it with the child (again, this depends on the age and maturity of the child).

The special needs of siblings of dying children must also be taken into consideration. They are often left out, while the dying child is spoiled with material things. Needless to say, these siblings grow extremely resentful, bitter, and jealous of the terminally ill child, although they would never want to change places with their brother or sister. This kind of behavior is frequently observed and can be prevented by an understanding counselor who encourages the parents not to overreact to their terminally ill child. Large quantities of material things, which the sick child neither needs nor really appreciates, do not relieve the parents of their sense of powerlessness at being unable to prevent or stop what their child is experiencing.

Dr. Stanford B. Friedman points out what he feels to be most important in helping the family deal with its situation: physicians should be consciously aware of the common modes of adjustment used by parents, for only in this way will health care professionals be able to anticipate their needs, problems, and sources of anxiety.[7] These professionals should be able to give the parents emotional and psychological guidance and recognize the diverse forms of "coping behavior" that parents often manifest through denial. It is very important that doctors demonstrate their willingness to answer all the parents' questions, that they clearly discuss the disease with the parents, and that they explain the various possible courses the illness could take. Participation by the parents in the child's care may also need to be guided; they may wish to stay with the child day and night in the hospital, or they may be reluctant to acknowledge how the child is feeling (denial). In either circumstance, the child must be part of all decision-making processes.

WHAT THE CHILD SHOULD BE TOLD

As has often been the case, the child is neglected when faced with a life-threatening illness. Much of the time and energy of the health care deliverer is spent helping the parents cope with the psychological upheaval of tending to a terminally ill child. Even though it is necessary to understand the problems of the parents, it is cruel to overlook the needs of the child.

In the past, it was believed that children could not understand the meaning of their illness, let alone be able to deal emotionally with its prospects if they were told. The results of further research have shown that children know the seriousness of their disease, and often the diagnosis, without being told directly. Surprisingly, sick children from as young an age as four may be aware of their illness. Since children do have such an accurate idea of the fate that approaches, the need to talk to them is even greater. The lack of discussion or acknowledgment to children regarding the seriousness of their illness may lead may the child to feel isolated or abandoned psychologically. Children believe that others are not aware of what they are experiencing, or even worse, they may feel that their disease is " too awful" to talk about.

It has been shown to be most beneficial to the children to make sure they know that both parents and physicians can answer their questions and are willing to discuss the sickness when the need arises. So, when first dealing with the child, it is important to establish a relationship that allows for questions, where it is understood that no barriers exist in discussing the topic of death. Children are capable of talking about death, and asking questions concerning their own death indicates that they really want to know.

There have been no established criteria as to how much to tell children but it is believed that the best method is to let them lead the way. When children feel comfortable and reassured, they will ask the questions that are most pertinent, and when satisfied with the information received, they will generally feel more at ease. It may take children weeks or even months to feel secure enough to ask the questions that most concern them, but it is important that the opportunity always exists for their questions to be asked and that they are always made aware of the willingness of parents and health care staff to answer any questions or discuss any topic.[8] When explaining the illness to the child, both physicians and parents should have a positive approach. The child responds much more to *how* something is said than to *what* is said. Thus the child is more impressed by the implied positive thinking conveyed by both the physician and parents. But physicians and parents should be cautioned not to oversimplify or relate the disease to a concept the child cannot fully comprehend. The best approach may be to draw the explanation as much as possible from the child's own experience. This allows for the least possible amount of distortion on the part of the child. To assure even further that the issue has not become more complicated by the explanations, it is a good idea to ask the child to restate in his own words what he has been told. This allows the adult to correct any misconceptions the child may have before they can cause any further damage.

A point that needs to be considered by both physicians and parents is that *children should be told of their diagnosis and its implications even if they don't ask for the information.* The reasoning behind this is that a child may be told by a playmate, which may cause serious emotional problems and distrust toward the physician or parents. If the illness is made known by adults, the child will at first cope with the news by denying the illness, but he will then be able to withstand any shock when told accidentally by a friend.[9]

CRISIS OF DISCOVERY

For parents, the crisis of discovery begins when they are first told the diagnosis of the fatal illness. No single event, with the exception of the child's death itself, has a greater impact on the life of a family. Many parents state that they had suspected that their child had a fatal disease before actually being told the diagnosis by the physician. Typically, parents respond by being stunned, shocked, or in a state of disbelief when hearing a definitive diagnosis. Most parents initially feel guilt and self-blame for not having paid more attention to the early, nonspecific manifestations of the disease. Many wonder if the child would have had a better chance of responding to therapy if the diagnosis had been made earlier. This self-blame is characteristically a transient phenomenon. More often, parents blame themselves for not having been more appreciative of the child before his or her illness. This attitude frequently leads to over-indulgence and over-protection of the fatally ill child, with no limits put on the child's behavior. Friedman interprets the shock as an extreme degree of isolation of affect, a mechanism by which the apparent intellectual recognition of a painful event is not associated with an accompanying intolerable emotional response. He reported that this lack of affective experience continued to be a conspicuous defense and enabled parents to talk realistically about their child's condition and prognosis with relatively little evidence of emotional involvement.[10] Typically, the dying child's grandparents tend to be less accepting of the diagnosis than the parents. More distant relatives and friends challenge the reality of the diagnosis even more frequently. Parents generally perceive most of these statements and suggestions as attempts to cheer them up and give them hope. Yet, parents often find themselves in the uncomfortable position of having to "defend" their child's diagnosis and prognosis. Sometimes the parents reported feeling that other people thought they were condemning their own child. Thus, these parents were not allowed to express any feelings of hopelessness, yet paradoxically they were expected to appear grief-stricken.

The reactions of children at the time of diagnosis depends upon a number of factors, including their age, what they are told about what is happening to them, and whether they are hospitalized. If their diagnosis is made during an acute episode of the disease, they may display little psychological response or open expression of emotion because their energies are being used in combating the disease process.

Richmond reported that, in the children he observed, rarely was there manifested overt concern about death. He interprets this as an attempt at psychological repression of anxiety concerning death. In general, his children seemed to have reacted with an air of passive acceptance and resignation. Associated with this often seemed to be an atmosphere of melancholia.[11] Although children may not understand the diagnosis, the prognosis, or the therapy, they are adept at reading messages and picking up clues and signals from those around them. Very young children perceive what is happening on an emotional level. Their parents are suddenly protective to the point of smothering them. Regression, temper tantrums, or various other forms of misbehavior may suddenly be allowed. Children as young as eight months of age have been observed reacting to their parents' emotional response to bad news.[12]

The home life of the family generally centers on the

terminally ill child. Both parents and siblings sacrifice time, money, and energy for the ill child. Parents admitted that the other children in the family were neglected during the illness. Social events are not enjoyed by the family, and parents feel guilty about being happy.

THE DYING TRAJECTORY

Discovery of a fatal disease marks the beginning of the dying trajectory. With diseases such as leukemia, this trajectory may extend three to five years, though some survive for even longer periods. Both the child and the family have to live with the ambiguities of an uncertain future. The adaptational tasks of these families require the parents to maintain an investment in the welfare and the future of the ill child, while at the same time knowing the terminal nature of their youngster's illness. The child needs to integrate the losses and changes produced by the illness, while continuing to fulfill whatever personal potential for life that still exists.

STAGES OF PSYCHOLOGICAL ADJUSTMENT

As Elisabeth Kübler-Ross noted, the process of learning to live with a fatal illness takes place in stages.[13] All of those involved, including family members, the child, and health care professionals go through a series of stages in which they assimilate the changes in the child's status into their own concept of reality. The first stage is shock and disbelief, during which denial is a commonly observed pattern of behavior. Anger or guilt and a gradual awareness of the change in the child's condition may occur next. One must reorganize relationships with other people, and one may attempt to strike a bargain with God to have death postponed. Resolution of the loss through active grieving must occur. There should also be reorganization and identity incorporating the loss of the loved one.

These stages do not necessarily take place in a certain order or in an easy manner. People generally have to repeat the stages each time the child goes through a serious episode of physical regression or hospitalization. People vary in their capacity to experience and openly display their anger, frustration, guilt, sadness, and grief. Persons who have been taught to openly express these emotions will usually move through the stages of psychological adaptation more easily than those who think of overt expression as a sign of weakness or loss of control.

AWARENESS OF DEATH

A problem of great concern for parents of a child with a fatal illness is how much the child knows, or should know, about the diagnosis and prognosis. According to Glaser and Strauss, the behavior of dying persons and their interaction with others is influenced by the "awareness context" in which they take place. An awareness context involves the degree of knowledge about a patient that one person has, in conjunction with that same person's perception of how much knowledge other involved people possess. The involved people will behave in a certain manner, based on how they perceive the others' degrees of knowledge.[14] As degrees of knowledge and acceptance vary, behavior patterns in the group will also change. For example, in one early awareness context, patients do not recognize their impending death, although everyone else does. The *suspected-awareness* context is a more advanced level which occurs when patients suspect what others know and attempt to confirm or negate their suspicions. In the *mutual-pretense* context, everyone defines the patient as dying, but each pretends that the others have not done so. In the *open-awareness* context, the patient and all of the others are aware that the death is imminent and express it openly.[15]

Glaser and Strauss stress that the impact of each type of awareness context influences the interaction among patient, family, and staff. Actions and conversations are guided by who knows what and with what degree of certainty. They argue that action, talk, and accompanying clues cause certain awareness contexts to develop into other contexts. This occurs when one of the persons in the interaction violates the rules necessary for maintaining that particular context. A new context then develops.

Advocates of the open-awareness approach argue that children with a fatal illness and their siblings need an environment in which they can ask questions and know what is happening. In such an environment, the parents give the child information about the illness and about the child's future. An awareness of impending death gives patients an opportunity to close their lives in the manner they wish. Open-awareness has disadvantages, too. Other people may not approve of the patients' way of managing their death and may attempt to change their ideas.

Bluebond-Langer's study revealed only two children who were able to develop an open-awareness context. The shift to open-awareness does not result from a breakdown in the mutual-pretense context. When open-awareness is achieved it is not necessarily final or complete in every area. There are lapses back to mutual-pretense when the child achieves a remission. Bluebond-Langer finds that parents of the children who have developed open-awareness are different from the children who practice mutual-pretense. These parents seem to derive most of their identity and sense of self-worth from sources other than the parental role. They are also more unconventional in their behavior and appear less concerned about society's judgment of their beliefs.

These parents also experience additional problems. They are sometimes ostracized by their peers for not protecting their child from the facts. Staff members appear not to be as helpful to these parents. The parents are also faced with more concrete problems of how to treat and what to say to the child. Yet, such parents of open-awareness children say that being honest with their child has helped them to cope with the prognosis. Honesty also has helped to bring them closer together.

Bluebond-Langer concludes that children practicing mutual-pretense and open-awareness behaved in the same manner. Both sets of children are preoccupied with death and disease imagery in their play, art, and conversation. They do not discuss going home and future plans, and they continue to practice distancing strategies.

Bluebond-Langer argues that the question is not

"Should I tell the child that he or she is dying?" but "Should I acknowledge the prognosis to the child?" She recommends that the needs of the child, family, and staff be taken into consideration. She recommends allowing the child to maintain open-awareness with those who can handle it and, at the same time, mutual-pretense with those who cannot. She suggests telling children only what they want to know, what they are asking about, and on their own level. The issue is not whether to tell children they are dying, but how to tell them in a way that respects them and their needs.

THE TERMINAL STATE

The terminal state is divided into three stages: the terminal phase, the terminal period, and the terminal event.

The Terminal Phase

The terminal phase may last weeks or months, but the general time frame is six months or less. The child may have frequent relapses, difficult remissions, and numerous complications. This phase marks a renewal of bargaining by both families and the patients themselves for experimental procedures, and finally for enough medication to relieve the child's pain.

Those involved with the dying child are often angry at this time. Parents may become angry if others talk about their child's future when it is so obvious that the child has none.

Children at this stage often lose interest in the outside world. They may become more depressed with each discharge from the hospital because they have accepted the painful reality that they can no longer participate in and enjoy the activities of family and friends. Older children know they will never get well and may wish that death would come. Rarely do older children resist until the end. Older children are usually resigned to their death before their family is and they often feel guilty because of this. Many children thank their parents for all they have done for them or ask forgiveness for the problems their illness has caused.

The Terminal Period

During the terminal period the inevitability of death is recognized and affirmed. Parents may say that they accept the inevitability of the child's death, but they do not always believe it. True acceptance means realizing that there is no hope for survival.

When death is near, the family may have to make a decision about whether the child will die at home. Decisions must also be made about possible organ donation and an autopsy.

Children in the terminal period of their illness will often, quite deliberately, stop talking about discharge, returning to school, or any future plans. They may become depressed or withdrawn. Some preschoolers with a perfect understanding of tenses have been noted to talk about their aspirations in the past tense.

Chinn reports that in some instances where parents

and children have experienced a very supportive and close relationship up to this point, they may mutually "recognize" the termination of further energy resources. Such children may begin to help their parents to stay away or to transfer their interest to other people and things. The children may find it too painful to watch their parents mourn. They may bid their parents good-bye too soon and may be left alone to die.[16]

The Terminal Event

The terminal event includes the hours preceding death itself. A child may rally before death and achieve a surprising alertness. Some parents regard this as a last treasured gift, others as a painful experience since they know so little time is left and there is so much to talk about.

Friedman reports that because of the anticipatory grieving which has already occurred, the child's death is generally taken calmly, but with the appropriate expressions of effect. Outbursts of uncontrollable grief or open expressions of self-blame are the exception. Usually there is some indication of relief that the child is no longer suffering. Friedman suggests that, therefore, the death of the child does not appear to be a severe, superimposed stressful situation but, rather, an anticipated loss at the end of a long sequence of events.[17]

CARE FOR CHILDREN WITH AIDS

Acquired immunodeficiency syndrome (AIDS) was first observed in homosexual men and intravenous drug users. Although it still remains a disease chiefly of these high-risk adults, today the fastest growing group of AIDS patients is not adults, however, but children. During the twelve-month period between 1987 and 1988, there were 416 cases of AIDS reported among children under the age of thirteen. This represents an increase of 85 percent over the total for the previous year.[18] To care appropriately for this growing AIDS population, we must consider the rights and responsibilities of society as well as of the patient.

There has been much hysteria concerning AIDS since the disease was first recognized in 1981. The presence of children with AIDS in schools has been the subject of intense emotional debate in a number of cities. An announcement in 1985 that an unidentified child with AIDS would be permitted to attend school led to several months of protests that resulted in a school boycott in one district and a court challenge.[19] Health care workers have also been reluctant to care for AIDS patients.

This hysteria concerning the disease is due largely to the misconception that the virus can be transmitted through casual contact. Although HIV has been isolated from blood, semen, saliva, tears, breast milk, and urine, epidemiological evidence has only implicated blood and semen in transmission. The virus can also be transmitted perinatally from mother to neonate.[20] The evidence against transmission through casual contact is mounting. In a study done of four hundred family members of adults and children with AIDS, no cases of household transmission were documented, except sexual partners of infected persons and children born to infected mothers. Epidemiological studies in the United States and countries throughout Europe suggest no patterns of HIV transmission related to insect bites.[21] Thus, fear about contracting the infection through casual contact is unjustified, and it is society's responsibility to provide care for AIDS patients comparable to that of any other terminally ill person.

Caring for the child with HIV represents a challenge for society. It requires the establishment of centers that are not only capable of providing care for the management of acute medical problems associated with AIDS and minimizing the immuno-suppressed child's exposure to infectious agents, but also skilled at providing social support to meet the psychosocial needs of patients and their families. Seventy-five percent of the HIV-infected children acquire their infections perinatally.[22] A study conducted at the Downstate Medical Center in Brooklyn, New York, suggests that women who deliver babies that develop AIDS are in significant medical and social jeopardy. In addition to having to care for a severely ill child, they themselves must be HIV-positive and at risk for developing the disease.[23] Should the mother's HIV-infection become full-blown AIDS, it is not inconceivable that such a child may require foster care.

Home care for the HIV-infected patient is quite feasible. The following are the only precautions issued by the Medical Society of New York to prevent acquisition of the virus during home care of infected patients:

Persons infected with HIV can be safely cared for in home environments. Studies of family members of patients infected with HIV have found no evidence of HIV transmission to adults who were not sexual contacts of the infected patients or to children who were not at risk for perinatal transmission. Health care workers providing home care face the same risk of transmission of infection as health care workers in hospitals and other health settings.

When providing health care service in the home to persons infected with HIV, measures similar to those used in hospitals are appropriate. As in the hospital, needles should not be recapped, purposefully bent, broken, removed from disposable syringes, or otherwise manipulated by hand. Needles and other sharp items should be placed in puncture resistant containers and disposed in accordance with local regulations for solid waste. Blood and other body fluids that cannot be flushed down the toilet should be wrapped securely in a plastic bag that is impervious and sturdy (not easily penetrated). It should be placed in a second bag before being discarded in a manner consistent with local regulations for solid waste disposal. Spills of blood or other body fluid should be cleaned with soap and water or household detergent. As in the hospital, individuals cleaning up such spills should wear disposable gloves. A disinfectant solution or a freshly prepared solution of sodium hypochlorite (household bleach) should be used to wipe the area after cleaning.[24]

Home care may in fact be the option of choice in many cases of pediatric HIV infections. In instances where children have been identified as HIV-infected, but do not yet manifest acute symptoms, they should be allowed to continue to experience a normal childhood. They should not be denied their educational rights. This, however, may present a problem. The diagnosis of AIDS still evokes fear. Many people still wrongly believe that the virus can be transmitted through casual contact. People who are suspicious of the lifestyles of HIV-infected children should be made aware of the potential for ostracism if the child's condition became known in an educational setting. Should such isolation became a reality, the health care team (doctors, nurses, social workers, and parents) must be prepared to discuss the problems with the afflicted child openly. This is of particular importance since the child's frustrations would be compounded if he or she were unable to find an outlet for discussing frustrations.

If the acute symptoms can be controlled without hospitalizing the child, home care for the AIDS patient would be economically sound. Twenty-five dollars per day is the average cost of home care for the dying child. Hospital care costs, on the other hand, range from $200 to $411.

Family members of AIDS patients often request counseling and support to help them accept the diagnosis and to deal with their own fears and to learn to be supportive. Grieving loved ones often need support in their bereavement. Mothers of children born with HIV infections need counseling to cope with their fears that they and their children may develop AIDS. Since the diagnosis of AIDS upsets the equilibrium of the whole family unit, it is necessary to provide care for the whole family. This sort of patient-family care is provided to terminal cancer patients at Hospice New Haven. The goals of this hospice home program are as follows:

(1) To aid in reducing the burden of a traumatic life experience by sharing and meeting the expressed needs (physical, emotional, spiritual, and social) of the patient and family;

(2) To assist the patient in achieving and maintaining maximum independent living and dignity until death;

(3) To minimize the painful and damaging effects of the death of a family member upon the surviving family members.

Much can be learned about providing care service for terminally ill patients and their families from Hospice New Haven. The service is individually tailored to meet the diverse patient-family needs. This model can be used to design care systems for people with AIDS and support for their families.

There is a need for health professionals who are familiar with all aspects of HIV infection. Health professionals from physicians to nurse's aides to social workers must acquaint themselves with medical, psychosocial implications of HIV infection such as depression, anxiety, hostility, loss of self-esteem, anger, acceptance, or denial. They must work together in order to care for the infected individual properly.

The prognosis for pediatric AIDS is poor; over 60 percent of the children diagnosed with AIDS die within six months.[25] The care of children with AIDS should be directed at reducing the number of people who contract HIV and AIDS. Therapeutic interventions should be directed at reducing discomfort and not unnecessarily prolonging a life with little quality. Thus care for the patient with AIDS requires not only tertiary care management of acute medical problems associated with HIV infection, but also social support skilled at meeting the psychosocial needs of the patients and their families. Since the number of children with AIDS is increasing, there is an urgent need to provide health care facilities that will meet the demands of this growing patient population. By adopting the holistic goals of the hospice home care program, which for over fourteen years has been providing care for the terminally ill cancer patient, we can begin to apply the humanistic care needed by AIDS patients who have only a little time left to enjoy life. Let's not waste this time of theirs by ignoring the fact that they are still living.

QUESTIONS AND ANSWERS FROM PARENTS

This section grew out of discussions among a number of parents who have survived one or more of their children. The life span of these parents' children ranged from forty days to fourteen years. They died from cystic fibrosis, heart defects, heart attacks, leukemia, and cancerous tumors. Although the ages of the children and the causes of their deaths varied, all the parents had the following concerns and questions in common.

Diagnosis

Diagnosis was the most difficult experience for most parents during the child's illness. They all asked: *"Why?"*

Why me? Why my child?" Most of the parents realize that they may never have an answer. Perhaps for some of the parents the growth they and their children experienced, and the lives that were softened and touched by children, are part of the answer.

"Am I going crazy? Is this normal?"

Parents frequently had these thoughts following the shock and pain of diagnosis. As they all felt numb and shocked and "crazy" for a while, this reaction seems to be "normal." All of them had a sense of being in a dream, and as one mother said, "I felt like I was watching [a medical drama] on TV." The parents wanted to be told of the diagnosis in some private area of the treatment center.

Medical Treatment

"Is my doctor doing all he can do for my child? Is he truthfully answering my questions? Is he explaining tests to me and to my child?"

Most of the parents had positive experiences with doctors and other medical personnel, but unfortunately, all of them had negative experiences as well. They felt anger and frustration when questions were ignored or were answered condescendingly. They saw their children treated as objects—as bodies with disease—by some (although there were compassionate people as well). Overwhelmingly, parents asking these questions urge others to speak up and ask their doctors for information. Fathers tended to be more assertive and many mothers expressed regret over past timidity. Insist that explanations be given to your child as well, no matter how young. As has been said earlier, given the proper context to fit the child's ability and willingness to know, any child can be informed of the diagnosis and the progress of care. Most parents felt that their doctors did their best, did all they were capable of doing.

Parents urge others to accompany their child during treatments and tests and to insist upon being allowed to do this. The children were less frightened and at least had a hand to hold. Also, children cannot speak up for themselves, so their parents act as valuable advocates. More than one parent has had to insist on a new nurse after watching repeated unsuccessful attempts to insert an intravenous needle.

Parents also encourage others to follow their intuition, their feelings. One mother described her gut feeling that something was seriously wrong when her pediatrician dismissed her daughter's swollen eyes as an allergic reaction (the child died of acute leukemia a few months later). The same mother described trying to stop a nurse from an unnecessary sample-gathering procedure likely to cause hemorrhaging. The nurse insisted and indeed did start a dangerous hemorrhage. Parents can avoid much anger and frustration by finding a doctor who will take their concerns seriously. Parents (mothers especially) can avoid guilt and anguish later by following their intuition.

"Did we fail to detect the early signs? What were the signs? What could we have done? How does the disease start? Would the outcome have been different if we'd known earlier?"

Unfortunately, many of the early signs of some of the children's fatal diseases were similar to the symptoms of less serious illnesses. Intermittent fevers, stomach aches, and listlessness can look like a cold or the flu. Runny, puffy eyes and nose can look like an allergy. The list is endless. Again, parents are urged to follow their intuition. You know your child best and you know when your youngster is behaving differently. But even with all these observations, it is often difficult to catch the early signs of a disease. The doctors often had a difficult time with diagnosis; parents with no medical experience were unlikely to detect early signs. The children often had diseases and treatments totally unfamiliar to their parents. We just don't know how many of these diseases start, and as yet have no way to prevent them. The parents all loved their children and tried to provide the healthiest diet and environment they could for them before and after illness. What better preventive medicine could there be?

Perhaps events would have been different if detection were early enough, but as one mother remarked, "not necessarily."

When the disease is hereditary there is a temptation for parents to blame each other, which adds to the pain of an already stressful event. It took both parents to produce the child and the possibility of disease had to be carried by both. Parents with children stricken with a hereditary disease did not know that they were carriers and in many cases had never heard of the disease before.

"Can it happen again?"

Young parents who wish to have more children are

especially plagued by this question. When the disease is clearly hereditary the question is answered, but when the disease is not considered hereditary the possibility remains. One couple, whose child died of a heart defect, were assured the condition was not hereditary, only to have another child who also died as a toddler from the same condition. Many felt concern that the disease might show up later in healthy siblings. There are no answers, but there are statistics that indicate the likelihood of a disease being hereditary, or of showing up in other family members. Again, do not be shy. Ask! If you are not satisfied with answers, ask the doctor to recommend some literature on the topic that you can read.

Coping

"Is there another parent I can talk to who is going through this? Is there another child my child can relate to?"
    Most of the parents went through their child's illness and death without knowing there were other families going through a similar experience. Many of them did not meet another bereaved parent until long after their child's death. All of them, and their dying children, would have liked knowing others. So many felt hopelessly alone. If there is a Center for Attitudinal Healing in your area, ask about parents' and children's groups. If not, ask the nurse or social worker for suggestions. Even if there is no Center for Attitudinal Healing near you, you can still apply for a phone/pen pal for you or your child.

"What helped you cope?"

Many parents were helped by religious faith and supportive friends. Some parents stressed knowledge about the disease as a coping factor. Reading about the condition, researching experimental methods, and learning about treatments available helped some parents endure their child's illness. They felt this might make the disease less foreign to them.

Most parents had to learn some treatment procedures to be followed at home (postural drainage for children with cystic fibrosis, for example). For some this was welcome, because it was something positive the parents could do, which made them feel less helpless.

Both parent and child needed to be able to make choices whenever possible and to maintain some control over the situation. This helped them feel less powerless and less helpless. Even the youngest children needed options. Making choices and having their wishes respected allowed them to feel needed.

"How does a single parent cope?"

It isn't easy, but it can be done. All of the single parents in this group were mothers, and all had financial problems which necessitated signing up for food stamps and other forms of state or government support. In some cases the child's father did participate in decision making and also in care, the latter usually on weekends. In several cases, the father was also present at the child's death. Even with the difficulties and stress of single parenthood, the mothers were able to care for their children at home, and with the cooperation of medical professionals and friends, some were able to have their children die at home also.

Family and Friends

"How can family and friends help? Should parents accept help? What advice can parents give so that friends and relatives can help constructively?"

There are so many ways to help. There is a role for everyone, and although all are not suited by temperament to give the child direct care, there are still many services the family needs. If you have a neighbor or friend who offers help and you feel comfortable with that person, accept the person's help and thank him for his concern. Give choices. Perhaps you have a small list of needs: help with siblings while you care for the sick child or visit at the hospital, grocery shopping, errands, helping with the housework or preparing meals, picking up prescriptions. If it is someone the child is comfortable with, you can accept help with the child's care and perhaps take a break yourself.

Friends and relatives can help best by tactfully accepting the situation. All of the parents received unnecessary though well-meaning advice. Sometimes people do have helpful suggestions, but they must offer them tactfully, remaining mindful of how emotionally vulnerable the parent of a very sick child can be. Friends and family can also help by refraining from adding burdens; this is not the time to recite woes and complaints. The parents are preoccupied with their own concerns.

Preparation for Death

"How will my child die? Is my child dying? Is my child afraid?"

Every parent needed to know what was likely to happen at the end. None of them had experience with a dying person before and they wanted to know what to expect. Some parents read about their child's disease and learned what to expect, but most wanted to ask questions. In almost every case the doctors were evasive in dealing with parents who normally had comfortable relationships with their doctors and had found them previously willing to answer questions. Most parents' questions were answered more satisfactorily by social workers or nurses. Parents wanted to know as soon as possible when their child was dying. Any early information they could obtain about the changes that were likely to occur in their child's condition lessened their fear.

Parents who were able to communicate openly with their children (what has been called open-awareness) learned from them not to fear death and in turn learned that the child was not afraid. This was true with a child as young as a two-and-a-half, whose mother reported that the little girl comforted her older sister with, "It'll be all right" and told her mother that she wanted "to go home." From songs the child sang, the mother understood that by "home" the child meant the dimension to which she would go to at death.

Death

"Will I authorize life-support systems? What will dying be like? Can parents be there while their child dies? Can they hold their child?"

None of the parents decided to prolong their child's life once it was apparent that the body could no longer function on its own. Older children requested that their parents not use life-support systems.

In some way all of the parents felt that they had "let go," that they gave their child permission to die. Each parent had to find some acceptance inside in order to let the child go. This did not negate the grief, but allowed them to experience some measure of peace at the death.

They were all present at the deaths of their children, and although the breathing sounds of the dying were foreign to them, they were grateful to be there and felt peace and relief, especially if the child had been suffering. It was comforting to them to see their children without life support, to see their faces uncluttered by oxygen masks or other apparatus. They all needed and wanted some quiet time alone with their child's body. For some it was the first opportunity in a long while to hold their child.

When death occurred at home, the parents had no difficulty getting time alone with their youngster, but when death occurred in the hospital, sometimes the parents were forced to insist on this. One couple watched the violent attempts to revive their ten-month-old from a heart attack and had to insist on remaining in the room, although nurses suggested they wait in the lobby. Then the father requested that he and his wife have time alone with their baby. The mother felt at peace holding her baby after the boy's ordeal. Both parents are thankful they had this time together with their son.

For most parents, this quiet time alone with their child was a peaceful interlude in the midst of the turmoil before and after their child's death. Some would have liked more time with the child's body and later regretted not having asked for it.

Many parents do not know that they are not required to have an autopsy performed on the child's body unless special circumstances require it. Part of a hospital's accreditation is based on the number of autopsies performed, so doctors ask, but parents do not have to consent. Also, if the funeral home has a refrigeration room, parents are not compelled by law to have the body embalmed (although there may be variations from state to state). These are things parents are not told unless they ask.

Grief

"Will the grieving parent ever be happy again? Can the family ever have good times again? What was the meaning of the child's life? Will the grief ever go away?"

All the parents went through intense grief after their child's death. The years pass, and most of these people are eventually able to have good times with their families again. Many times they are grateful to have had the child at all, if only for a little while. Had any of them known of the pain and suffering they and their child would go through, and had they been able to prevent their child's birth, they all say they still would have chosen to have their child. The parents learned so much from their children (when they let the child teach them) and saw so many lives touched and deepened by them. They saw their children, even very young children, deepen and grow from their experience. Often their youthful wisdom was amazing. They gave their parents love and trusted them with their lives. The parents did the best they were capable of doing and felt grateful to their children for the time they had spent with them.

For most parents their children are still alive in some way. They are alive in the hearts of those who loved them. They live on in the lives they touched. They are alive in the totality of the cosmos, for as science tells us today, nothing is ever lost, just transformed. No particle of energy is extinguished, just converted. Those with a belief in an immortal soul feel that their child is still living and growing.

Suggestions

"What would the parents tell another parent going through this?"

Most parents emphasized the need to speak up and urge their peers not to be intimidated. Ask to read your child's medical record if you wish. (Most parents did want to, but didn't think it was allowed.) Question the treatments and procedures if you have doubts. Be honest with yourself and your child whenever you can.

Let yourself learn from your child. Forget once in a

while that you are the parent, the authority, and let yourself go through the experience with your child as a fellow student, both learning together.

"What would parents like to tell medical personnel and treatment centers?"

Remember that you are treating children, fragile human beings, not machines. Show your humanity. Give the child, no matter how young, some explanation of what you are doing. Your efficiency won't suffer if you relate to the child with a smile or a word. Remember that the child, no matter how old, may be frightened by machinery and tests, and this type of fear does not aid healing. Relaxation and trust promote healing, and you can help by making the event less fearful. Include the parents whenever possible.

Make your treatment area less grim. As one mother explained, "Even though the examinations weren't painful, my two-year-old son was very frightened when he had echocardiograms. If only there had been puppets or mobiles or something for him to look at during the test." Cheerful, soothing music could help too. These are not very expensive or time-consuming suggestions, but they could easily be incorporated by medical personnel.

Above all, take time to answer questions, even if you have answered them before. Many parents are under such stress that they may need further explanation. Neither you nor the parent are alone in wanting what is best for the child. You are working together for the child's well-being.

NOTES

1. M. Powazek, "Emotional Reactions of Children to Isolation in a Cancer Hospital," *Journal of Pediatrics* 92, no. 5 (1978): 836.

2. I. A. Martinson, "Home Care for Children Dying of Cancer," *Pediatrics* 62, no. 1 (1978): 108.

3. L. R. Samaniego, "Exploring the Physically Ill Child's Self-Perceptions and the Mother's Perceptions of Her Child's Needs," *Clinical Pediatrics* 19, no. 2 (1977): 157.

4. Lattanzi-Licht and S. Conner, "Care of the Dying: The Hospice Approach," in *Dying: Facing the Facts,* eds. H. Wass and R. Neimeyer (Washington, D.C.: Taylor & Francis, 1995), pp. 143–62.

5. Morris Green, "Care of the Child with a Long-Term, Life-Threatening Illness: Some Principles of Management," *Pediatrics* 39, no. 3 (1967).

6. Ibid.

7. S. B. Friedman, "Behavioral Observations of Parents Anticipating the Death of a Child," *Pediatrics* 32, no. 3 (1963).

8. Green, "Care of the Child."

9. G. P. Koocher, "Talking with Children about Death," *American Journal of Orthopsychiatry* 44, no. 3 (1974): 410.

10. S. Friedman et al., "Behavioral Observations of Parents Anticipating the Death of a Child," in *Counseling Parents of the Ill and the Handicapped,* ed. R. Nolan (Springfield, Ill.: Charles Thomas, 1971), pp. 458–74.

11. Cited in J. E. Gyulay, *The Dying Child* (New York: McGraw-Hill/Blakiston, 1978), p. 8.

12. B. Glaser and A. Strauss, *Awareness of Dying* (Chicago: Aldine de Gruyter, 1965), pp. 9–10.

13. Elisabeth Kübler-Ross, *On Death and Dying* (New York: Macmillan, 1969).

14. M. Bluebond-Langer, *The Private World of Dying Children* (Princeton, N.J.: Princeton University Press, 1978), pp. 200–22.

15. Ibid.

16. P. Chinn, *Child Health Maintenance* (St. Louis, Mo.: C. V. Mosby, 1974).

17. Friedman et al., "Behavioral Observations."

18. "Quarterly Report to the Domestic Policy Council on the Prevalence and Rate of Spread of HIV and AIDS in the United States," *Journal of the American Medical Association* 259, no. 18 (1988): 2657–61.

19. "Human Immunodeficiency Virus Infections in Children: Public Health and Policy Issues," *Pediatric Infectious Diseases Journal* 6 (1987): 113–16.

20. "Guidelines for the Protection of Health Care Workers in Caring for Persons Who Have Some Form of HTLV-III/LAV Infection," *New York Journal of Medicine* 86, no. 11 (n.d.): 587–91.

21. "The Epidemiology of AIDS in the U.S.," *Scientific American* 259 (n.d.): 72–81.

22. "Quarterly Report to the Domestic Policy Council."

23. "Pregnancies Resulting in Infants with Acquired Immunodeficiency Syndrome or AIDS-Related Complex: Follow-up of Mothers, Children, Subsequently Born Siblings," *Obstetrics and Gynecology* 69 (July/August 1988): 285–91.

24. "Guidelines for the Protection of Health Care Workers."

25. "Update on HIV Infection: Pediatric Aspects," *Maryland Medical Journal* 36, no. 1 (n.d.): 37–39.

7

Hospice Care for the Person with AIDS

As we have read, fear and AIDs run hand-in-hand. People are afraid of contracting the virus. Many think that they were safe if they do not participate in any "risk-taking" behaviors. Now, however, other issues have been brought to the surface regarding HIV. Health care workers, patients, physicians, and all other types of people are concerned. To settle some of these fears and to gain a better understanding of the issues, knowledge and education are needed.

Along with hospice and AIDS come many issues that need to be considered. The physicians' attitudes toward hospice are important, especially if they resist the concept. Health care workers' attitudes and ideas about persons with AIDS (PWAs) are very relevant. Another major issue is the screening of health care workers for

HIV. The role of both palliative and aggressive care in the hospice program and decision making for the continuance of care are two matters that often arise. And finally, the quality of life needs to be evaluated in both hospice and nonhospice settings.

PHYSICIANS' ATTITUDES TOWARD HOSPICE

Physicians are sometimes resistant to the concept of hospice. One reason underlying this resistance is the physicians' own attitude toward death. A study comparing physicians' fears of death with the fears of healthy and seriously (some terminally) ill patients revealed that physicians showed significantly more fear of death than either the healthy or sick lay people. While this fear seems today to be a factor in certain physicians' selection of medicine as a career, when modern medicine is looked upon as an aggressive *conquest* of death, it also may prevent them from being able to help patients deal with impending death.[1]

The physician's discomfort in this area of patient support is of relatively recent origin. Until forty years ago, cure was rare, and death was accepted as a natural consequence of having lived. The primary obligation of the physician was to bring comfort to the patient, whether that patient was going to get better or not. Now that medical science has learned how to cure far more effectively, death has come to be seen as unnatural and as the enemy of the physician.[2] Supported by the advanced medical training that has been in place since after World War II, and by their arsenal of antibiotics and other interventions, most physicians believe they can cure most diseases. They forget that most serious illness in this society results from chronic and not acute disease, and is therefore not amenable to seemingly magical technical interventions. Doctors believe overwhelmingly that the goal of their endeavors should be to cure and that anything less is failure.[3] Another reason for some physicians' resistance to hospice is that they see it primarily as a nursing function; or as a system of giving care rather than prescribing cure. When investigation, diagnosis, prolongation of life, and cure no longer seem relevant, physicians frequently conclude that they have nothing more to offer and therefore tend to remove themselves from the picture. However, a great deal remains for physicians to do for the dying person once cure is no longer a possibility.[4] They can help the patient cope with the frightening experience of the dying process. Patients fear the indignity of bodily degeneration, which includes loss of bowel control, offensive odors, disfiguring lesions, dependence on others, pain, suffocation, dementia, and abandonment. Competent and caring physicians can explain the course of the illness clearly to patients and can anticipate problems to allow for early intervention. They can also assist patients in gaining some measure of control over their lives by teaching them the proper use of medications and other ways to remain in charge of their health.[5]

More and more physicians are referring PWAs to hospice programs. While this is often an appropriate action, there is a potential danger that their frustration with being unable to cure these persons may lead them to make the referral too soon.[6]

ATTITUDE OF HEALTH CARE WORKERS TOWARD PWAs

Working with persons with AIDS presents many difficulties for health care workers. First of all, since those suffering from the disease are mostly young men and women in their thirties and forties, young doctors and nurses have to deal with the issue of identifying and coming to terms with their own vulnerability and mortality. For physicians in particular, this compounds their great fear of death.

Fear of transmission of the deadly disease is also common among health care workers. While the risk is low and measures exist to further reduce that risk, accidental injury and infection is certainly possible.[7] In the summer of 1987, the Centers for Disease Control (CDC) reported that three health care workers who were splashed with HIV-seropositive blood became infected with HIV. This manner of exposure had not previously been thought to be a hazard. Other researchers demonstrated that occupational transmission of HIV would not be limited to being accidentally stuck with AIDS-infected needles. Consequently, health care workers began to file suits. Furthermore, physicians and other health care workers began refusing surgery to PWAs and limiting the care they might receive. As a result of this fear on the part of the health community, HIV-seropositive individuals may have difficulty receiving the medical attention they need.

Health administrators must be sensitive to the fears of the health care workers in their institutions. It is not helpful to cite statistics to an individual who has slashed his hand while doing a spinal tap on a woman with a history of intravenous-drug use or to someone else who is experiencing symptoms that might be AIDS-related. Administrators should also ensure that they are following all recommended procedures for the protection of their workers. Even so, workers' professional and moral obligations toward the patients they serve must be made clear to them.

CASE STUDY

A twenty-nine-year-old man with severe classic hemophilia came to a local hospital because he felt very dizzy and fainted each time he stood. The hospital knew him well since he had a seven-year history of HIV infection and AIDS-related syndromes. The emergency room triage nurse determined that this was not an emergency and left him in the waiting room for four hours. The patient, not having the physical strength to protest, was finally seen by an intern. Even though the patient was severely anemic, the intern delayed treatment for at least an hour after examining him. The resident in charge of the emergency room knew the patient had low blood pressure and was a hemophiliac, but did not treat him as a critically ill case.

Ordinarily that patient's symptoms would be suggestive of a gastrointestinal hemorrhage, yet no attempts were made to consider treating the bleeding diuresis (an increase urine outflow containing blood) early on. Perhaps, consciously or subconsciously, this usually competent and energetic team decided to treat this patient differently because he had AIDS.[8]

SCREENING OF HEALTH CARE WORKERS

The public's fear of being infected by a seropositive care-giver has been an issue for some time now. This fear has led some to demand that health care workers be tested. In August 1987, the CDC stated that up to that point, there had been no reports of transmission of HIV from infected health care workers to patients. It did point out, however, that transmission during invasive proce-dures remained a possibility.[9] A recent investigation by the CDC found it likely that a Florida dentist, Dr. David J. Acer of Stuart, had transmitted HIV to three of his pa-tients. The dentist has since died.[10] Among the more than 160,000 cases of AIDS reported since the initial outbreak in 1981, these are the only known incidents in which the disease was probably transmitted from a health care worker to a patient.

Many questions are raised by this issue, not the least of which being: should caregivers be tested? In closing a two-day meeting that discussed the risk of transmis-sion of HIV from doctors and dentists to their patients, Dr. William Roper, head of the CDC, affirmed that, in the opinion of most, the mandatory testing of health care workers for AIDS was neither necessary nor useful. (He did not, however, discuss whether health care work-ers already infected with AIDS should be required to in-form their patients.) The consensus at the meeting focused on the need for greater application of infection-control procedures and continued research to develop better and safer equipment in order to protect both pa-tients and health care workers, including the issuance of new guidelines to protect patients against transmission of the AIDS virus from health care workers.[11]

The wisdom of mandatory testing of all health care workers does indeed seem questionable. While it is true that three patients seem to have been infected by a health care worker, this rare occurrence cannot be used to justify the invasive and costly enterprise such a testing program would involve. And while transmission of the hepatitis B virus (HBV), a blood-borne agent with a considerably greater potential for spreading from health care workers to patients, has been documented, that mode of infection has occurred only during the performance of certain types of invasive procedures. Strict adherence to infection-control measures will result in minimal risk of transmission. If such testing is ever put in place the same principles of testing that are used in testing programs of patients should govern this program. Those principles are:

(1) Consent should be obtained.

(2) The worker must be informed of the results and counseling must be provided for that person.

(3) Confidentiality must be assured so that the knowledge is limited to those with a need to know.

(4) There must be an evaluation of the efficacy of the program in reducing the incidence of infection of patients by health care providers and of the effect of the procedure on the health care worker.[12]

A serious consideration of the fourth principle might lead to the conclusion that such a program is not useful or cost-effective.

The question remains: Should health care providers who are seropositive be allowed to practice, or should they be discharged or limited in their practice? Since health care institutions have not formulated a stable policy, the relatively few employees whose cases have come to the institutions' (and the public's) attention have been dealt with on a case-to-case basis.[13] Some fear that the new guidelines to be issued by the CDC could include proposals to restrict the practice of infected health care workers.[14] Such restrictions can only exacerbate the epidemic of fear already existing in the community. Furthermore, they may distract the medical community from the efforts it must make for infection control. And finally, such regulations would protect no one. The identified seropositive person would be restricted, while unidentified health care workers would be practicing without restriction. Such restrictions may impact on the health system with a deadly irony: they may effectively reduce the number of individuals willing to work with AIDS patients, since these restrictions would in effect eliminate from the field of clinical practice the very caregivers who might be most sympathetic to persons with AIDS. This would worsen an already serious shortage of health care workers available to provide necessary services to people with AIDS.[15]

PALLIATIVE CARE VERSUS AGGRESSIVE CARE

Should aggressive care be used in a hospice setting? With the hope for a cure ever present, there may exist an ambivalent attitude toward relinquishing treatment. Persons with AIDS often seek palliative therapy while simultaneously seeking curative therapy. Ongoing discussion among patients, physicians, nurses, and other team members is vital and should include when to stop curative therapy. The family, who is considered part of the unit of care, should also be involved in these discussions. However, the patient must be considered the key member of the team, deciding preferences for treatment, home or hospital management, and type and number of social interactions.[16] The rules of confidentiality would also dictate that the patient determines what information is shared with other, nonmedical, members of the team.

Even in the terminal phases, active interventions may be appropriate in some cases. One example is the early use of ganciclovir to prevent blindness resulting from retinitis caused by a herpes virus. The positive result of this therapy must be weighed against the trauma that accompanies it. The patient must have a central line inserted and have infusions two times per day for two weeks followed thereafter by infusions daily or several times a week. This curative therapy may be chosen by the patient either on his own or following consultation with members of the team. While all team members should provide their honest input, the final decision should be left to the patient.[17]

Persons with AIDS who dread the onset of HIV en-
cephalopathy (brain disease) have the possibility of taking oral zidovudine (AZT) which slows the spread of HIV,
consequently adding to the quality of their lives. Some
patients may choose to forego this active therapy because of the trauma of the regular blood transfusions
that are often required. While tests have shown that
AZT may extend a patient's life for more than a year,[18]
the patient will have to make the decision whether the
extra time gained by the treatment justifies the steps he
or she has to take to extend that life.

In the final analysis, while aggressive care may be
appropriate in some instances for persons with AIDS in
a hospice program, only palliative care is ultimately relevant.

CASE STUDIES

The first case illustrates the moment of decision for a patient whose life was being extended by blood transfusions. "Jim" had suffered from AIDS for thirteen months
and was in the last stages of the disease. He had one
devastating onslaught of pneumocystis carinii pneumonia and was thought to have Kaposi's sarcoma (KS) lesions in his esophagus, making swallowing very difficult.
The physician believed that these lesions were causing
the steady fall in Jim's blood count. Blood transfusions
no longer produced any noticeable improvement in his
energy level. On the day Jim died, he had requested one
more unit of red blood cells to give him energy over the
weekend. While waiting for the blood to arrive, he became increasingly nauseated and weak, and vomited

three cups of fresh blood, indicating an acute gastrointestinal bleeding. He and his hospice nurse discussed his next course of action. The hospice nurse told him he would most likely die in the next few hours if he did not go to the hospital for treatment of the active bleeding. He decided not to seek treatment and died that evening with his family and pastor at his bedside.[19]

The second case history is that of a thirty-five-year-old married mother of two employed as a secretary. She was diagnosed with an advanced malignant tumor of the upper chest wall and armpit with the presumed primary location of the cancer to have been in the breast. Two months later, the social worker from the palliative care team met her on an initial visit to the outpatient oncology clinic. The involvement of a member of the palliative care team at a point far before the terminal stage of illness allowed the professional caregivers to help her until she died. It also supported her right to make "care-or-cure" choices. The social worker helped not only the couple, but also their children in exploring how seriously ill the patient was. As her condition deteriorated, the various therapies that were attempted failed. The patient had uncontrollable movement of her left arm, increasing nausea and vomiting, and poor pain control. She had numerous medical interventions during their hospital stay. Decisions concerning those interventions were made through ongoing discussions among the patient, family, palliative care team, family physician, nursing staff, resident physicians, consultants, and housekeepers.

The team decided that it would be flexible as an interdisciplinary health service delivery team. Although some of her choices for intervention seemed inappropriate to the palliative care team and others appeared poor choices to the oncology team, everyone supported her right to make those decisions. They included the patient remaining in the hospital when she was physically able to be home, her choice of drugs to take for relief of symptoms, and which blood tests to have. The group supported her when she brought in outside drugs and herbal cures.

A week before she died, the patient was angry "that there were no treatments left." She managed all her medications, including ones for pain. Only on the morning of her death did she release management of her treatment plan and allow the team to decide what was best for her. The team had acted in this way because they wanted to give her the choice to live her own life until she died.[20]

DECISION MAKING FOR CONTINUANCE OF CARE

Another issue for discussion is the decision about responding to an "untreatable condition" such as respiratory failure. Who will make the decision whether or not to put the patient on a life-support system? This issue is particularly difficult in cases where the person with AIDS is no longer competent because of a neuropsychological condition. If the unit of palliative care is the family, who should be considered "family"? If the AIDS patient is living with a lover, who can make this type of decision in the absence of a durable power of attorney?[21]*

---

*A "power of attorney" is a written statement authorizing a person to act on another's behalf. In the example given, the AIDS patient would have such a document drawn up designating his lover as the person with the authority to decide what measures may be taken.

It seems that the right time to reach these decisions is early on in the course of the disease, when the patient is capable of participating. A "living will" should be considered. However, this is not done in many cases, since health care providers are reluctant to discuss such an issue with new patients when they are still well. The problem is compounded by the fact that the patient population is young (average age is twenty-eight to thirty-four), highly intelligent (with an average length of sixteen years of formal education in the first ten thousand U.S. cases), and often from strongly artistic backgrounds. Young women and children are also affected. It is difficult or impossible to discuss this kind of issue with what some caregivers consider "sympathetic" victims such as hemophiliacs, other blood transfusion-related cases, and babies. All these factors make discussion about the future course of treatment problematic.[22]

CASE STUDY

"Frank," a thirty-six-year-old man, was told that his doctor suspected AIDS after Frank had complained of specific symptoms—fatigue for about six months, diarrhea for four weeks, and some difficulty with concentration. Frank had admitted to his family physician that he was gay and that he had a stable five-year relationship with Bill. Frank was ultimately diagnosed with pneumocystis carinii pneumonia. Further testing showed moderate cognitive impairment. When the hospital decided that more tests were necessary, medical personnel were not sure who was empowered to give consent to the planned investigations, since Frank himself was unable to give informed consent.

Frank's parents, Susan and Paul, who were aware of their son's sexual orientation, had had little contact with him over the past few years. When the medical team contacted them, they appeared at the ward nearly in shock and gave consent for further testing. There followed discussion of who would care for Frank since he could not care for himself. Although Frank's lover insisted that Frank had wanted him to care for his needs, there was no documentation to support this position.

Frank's parents urged that they should take care of their son in his last days. Frank was unable to express any clear thoughts on this matter due to his cognitive impairment. The only sign of his intention was that he moved his chair close to Bill during one of the discussions. The palliative care physician, who met with all of them, helped them reach a mutually acceptable decision. Frank would stay with Bill in their apartment. Susan and Paul would provide some help in looking after Frank two or three days a week while Bill went to work to look after his business. Frank was subsequently hospitalized on two occasions. He died peacefully at home three months later.[23]

QUALITY OF LIFE: HOSPICE VERSUS NONHOSPICE CARE

Does hospice as a model of terminal care achieve the outcomes claimed by its proponents? Is there a difference between hospice and nonhospice patients' quality of life? According to a comprehensive survey of literature on this issue made by Vincent Mor, the dimensions of quality of life that were measured in various studies included pain, symptoms, physical quality of life, satisfaction with care, patients' psychosocial outcomes, where patients die, and family members' outcomes (both psychosocial and health-related). Let us examine these factors individually.

The studies showed that hospice clearly does not result in patients experiencing increased pain. In fact, some comparisons report that hospice may achieve small but significant improvements in pain control. The improvements were observable only when the base rates of pain in the study population were relatively high and when information was received from observers rather than from the patients, since they were often too sick to report on their own condition.

Hospice claims that the severity of symptoms, such as difficulty in breathing, nausea, and vomiting, as well as indicators of cognitive functioning, might be affected by hospice. The results in the literature concerning the comparison of the level of symptoms in hospice and nonhospice patients were mixed. There were also varying results concerning the level of cognitive functioning. There is still insufficient evidence that hospice is more effective than conventional care in controlling patients' physical symptoms and maintaining patients' awareness of their surroundings.

Overall quality of life refers to both physical and psychosocial functioning. The studies concluded that quality of life relating to physical functioning does not appear to be affected, either for good or ill, by hospice. Those findings concerning psychosocial functioning were even more ambiguous.

Patients served in hospices were more satisfied, overall, with the care that they received when compared to nonhospice patients. This positive effect, however, may be associated only with the inpatient variety of hospice. The studies also found that although the families of home-care patients were satisfied, they were not significantly more satisfied than were nonhospice patients' families. In general, however, hospice does appear to provide to the patients and the families the kind of service that they want. They have fewer regrets about the orientation of the care received than do nonhospice patients.

The studies focusing on patient psychosocial outcomes seem to indicate that the hospice philosophy does not have the indirect effect on the patients' psychological status at which hospice aims. The evidence suggests that explicit psychosocial intervention can work, at least under optimal conditions. The problem in the ultimate analysis may be financial. Will these programs be able to pay for the integration of psychosocial and medical services?

Hospice does facilitate arrangements for dying at home for those patients and families desiring it, whereas the nonhospice system does not. There were differences in the likelihood of death at home between the hospice program emphasizing home care and the hospices with inpatient units. In the program that emphasized home care, between 30 percent and 70 percent of patients died at home. In the inpatient units, between 20 percent and 30 percent did. The hospice movement allows for choice, since death at home is not necessarily to be desired in all cases.

Studies of the impact of the programs on the family's

anxiety and depression while the patient was living produced contradictory findings. One study found primary care persons in hospital-based hospices to be more satisfied with the care then primary care persons in conventional care situations. This may be due to hospice families feeling more involved in the care. In a home care setting, however, the involvement often becomes so intense that the family ends up feeling burdened.

Bereavement affects people's health. Indeed, the grief of bereavement can seriously affect those with preexisting health problems. Studies of the effects of hospice bereavement counseling has resulted in mixed findings, which may be due to the fact that a high proportion of people not really in need of counseling were included in the studies. Also, every hospice defines bereavement services differently. The literature seems to indicate that only a minority of bereaved persons benefit from intervention. It also appears that the most effective programs are those that are professionally administered with interpersonal contact over several months and those that are targeted only to the people who really need the counseling.[24]

CARES AND CONCERNS

The care of the acutely ill person with AIDS requires the most skillful application of nursing knowledge. Many of the guidelines for the care of patients with AIDS parallel those for the patients with other pulmonary, neurologic, oncologic, and systemic diseases. However, unlike these patients, persons with AIDS often experience more adverse reactions to medications and present special challenges because of lifestyle issues related to their diseases and care.[25] When caring for people with AIDS, one must realize that they are carrying a lot of "baggage," including rejection, isolation, hostility, depression, denial, and anger. Those working with this population must be aware of these factors in order to be effective in administering care. The nurse, being a very important person in the life of the person with AIDS when in the hospital, should provide an atmosphere of individual acceptance of the patient. This means putting aside one's personal feelings or prejudices about the patient's lifestyle or background. Because of the nurse's intimate contact with the patient, the person with AIDS quickly discovers whether the nurse is bringing a personal agenda to the bedside. The nurse should provide the patient with opportunities to express the strong feelings being experienced during this crucial time.

Anxiety and fear, combined with anger and depression, are often seen in the newly hospitalized AIDS patient. This anxiety may stem partially from not having a specific diagnosis; however, it can also be related to the patient's self-image, since AIDS, like many diseases, can alter one's self-concept.

The terminal stage of AIDS is not well defined. Although life expectancy after diagnosis remains approximately two years, patients have a wide variety of clinical options. Many die during a first acute hospitalization for pneumocystis carinii pneumonia. A final phase of irreversible decline is marked by successive, uncontrollable, opportunistic infections, progressive general deterioration and debilitation, and often deteriorating mental capacity.[26]

The onset of dementia, successive or multiple opportunistic infections, or irreversible debilitation may signal the need to consider a shift in the focus of treatment from aggressive, active diagnosis and intervention to a palliative approach designed to allow the patient to die in dignity and comfort. AIDS is a miserable disease. Those afflicted with it know that they are going to die. Therefore, in discussing cares and concerns, we are talking about *where* persons with AIDS will receive care, *what type* of care will be provided, *who* will provide care, and *what* the concerns are of those providing care to these terminally ill persons.

Arranging appropriate care for the terminally or chronically and progressively ill AIDS patient can be a challenge. However, in contrast with the typical scenario in a terminal disease such as cancer, multiple opportunistic complications and central nervous system impairment may cause AIDS patients to need intensive, twenty-four-hour-a-day personal care and supervision for months before death. The comprehensive approach of hospice care at home is increasingly seen as a model for treatment of patients entering the chronic, progressive, or terminal stages of AIDS.[27] The goal of hospice care for people with AIDS is to assist the client and family to achieve optimal function and obtain comfort despite the patient's progressive physical and often mental deterioration.[28] But this becomes a special challenge given the unpredictability and severity of the AIDS assault.

Hospice programs that are bound to traditional admission criteria of life expectancy, palliative care, and a primary support system are struggling to admit and care for people with AIDS. Hearing of and experiencing these limitations on admission, people with AIDS often resist being admitted and cared for by hospice programs. By the same token hospices—traditionally committed to patients whose life expectancy is six months or less, and for whom curative or aggressive therapy has been discontinued—cannot accurately predict life expectancy of AIDS patients at a time when intense research is under way to devise and evaluate new drugs and treatment strategies.[29] One of the critical requirements for working with the person with AIDS is the worker's availability, reliability, empathy, and ability to respond emotionally to the client, particularly during times of decline. The stress placed on the professional by such expectations cannot be overemphasized.[30]

Dunkel and Hartfield have identified eight countertransference issues associated with the care of the person with AIDS. These include fear of the unknown, fear of contagion, fear of dying and death, denial or helplessness, homophobia, over-identification, anger, and the need to profess omnipotence.[31] As the client nears death, these issues may intensify for the hospice staff. Because of the increasing number of AIDS patients, staff can become emotionally overwhelmed with little time to process and reintegrate. One staff member speaks from personal experience:

> AIDS puts a hospice nurse at risk for burnout because there seems to be no predictable course, and the usual methods and treatments that are helpful for cancer patients often do not work for AIDS. In my practice, most of my tried-and-true interventions are not successful. Very little of what I have done or know apply to AIDS

except, perhaps, the ability to hang in there until the end—and most of the time I am doing so by only the thinnest thread. The many tricks I have cultivated for hospice patients do not work well with AIDS patients, leaving me feeling frustrated and alone.[32]

Wallace outlines five guidelines that will enable hospice caregivers to cope more effectively with the problems associated with caring for patients with AIDS:

(1) Clarify for AIDS patients and their loved ones what hospice *cannot* do for them before specifying what it *can* do.

(2) Keep your professional footing. Because hospice personnel are usually close in age to AIDS patients and their loved ones, it is easy to over-identify and thus to become enmeshed in patients' struggles to live and die with AIDS.

(3) Learn to listen to your own feelings of helplessness and frustration.

(4) Speak the unspeakable in order to disengage various conflicting values and emotions in the patient-family unit.

(5) Get in touch with your own fears about AIDS— fears of contagion, death at a young age, homosexuality, and the drug culture.[33]

Wallace also suggests that by far the most serious and difficult obstacle blocking hospice care for AIDS patients is the lack of primary care persons in the home.

Clark and associates have identified AIDS dementia in particular as one of the most difficult complications of this disease to manage at home. Nursing care includes the provision of memory cues; behavioral modification, and the creation of a safe and predictable environment.

WHY HOSPICE?

Changes in reimbursement by health insurance plans are mandating shorter hospital stays. Prospective payments, which originally affected only Medicare patients, are rapidly being expanded to apply to all insurers for all patients. Because of this, hospices have moved into the mainstream of the health care system. The Joint Commission on Accreditation of Hospitals has developed comprehensive standards for the accreditation of hospice programs. Blue Cross/Blue Shield, Medicare, Medicaid, and most other major third-party payers provide benefits for hospice care. A major rationale for hospice reimbursement by Medicare and other insurance programs is the premise that hospice care, by substituting home-care services for hospital inpatient care, is less expensive than conventional care.[34]

In hospice, the unit of care is the entire family, and mandated benefits include the services of physicians, nurses, social workers, and other health professionals in the home, hospital, or nursing home; medication for pain relief and symptom control; medical appliances and equipment; nutrition counseling; extensive health and support services in the home; and bereavement counseling for the patient's family for up to one year.[35]

The hospice philosophy seems well suited to care for people with AIDS, especially with the use of a multidisciplinary team. Since no one professional can deal with every issue confronting the patient, the team tends to diffuse the intensity of effort in order not to overwhelm any one individual.

The AIDS Home Care and Hospice Program, a program of visiting nurses and hospice of San Francisco, used a multidisciplinary team of nurses, social workers, attendants, and volunteers available on a twenty-four-hour basis in consultation with each patient's primary physician. Some people with AIDS lack any support system. To allow the patient to stay at home, hospice team members may assume this responsibility, including:

- pain and symptom management

- emotional support

- a multidisciplinary care team

- pastoral/spiritual counseling

- bereavement counseling

- twenty-four-hour, on-call nurse or counselor

- staff support

People with AIDS thus feel secure in the knowledge that there is someone to call on an around-the-clock basis. Remaining at home while comforting, can be isolating as well. Crises often occur at night or on weekends when it is more difficult to contact support systems. Having an on-call nurse to offer advice by telephone or to make a home visit helps to reduce anxiety. Pain may not be as much of a concern for the AIDS patient as diarrhea or difficulty in breathing. The hospice approach emphasizes symptom control and the use of treatments or medications that allow the person to live comfortably.

QUALITY OF CARE

A multidisciplinary team approach entails a comprehensive effort to deal with the patients' medical, social, psychological, and spiritual problems over a period of time and in a variety of settings. These are among the important objectives of a program for the care of the terminally ill. The benefits of a multidisciplinary approach derive from the diversity of talent it brings to the task, but it is most vulnerable in its need for coordination among team members. An important feature of multidisciplinary care in a hospice program is the lack of a sharp distinction among the functions of various team members. Although each has expertise and primary responsibility, each must also be alert to the problems and needs of the patient in other areas.

Caring for the person with AIDS or AIDS-Related Complex (ARC) is an unprecedented challenge for those providing home hospice care. Those with AIDS, however, benefit immeasurably from the multidisciplinary approach adopted by most hospice programs. Indeed, the physical and psychosocial complexities of AIDS require this sensitive and humane approach.[36] Although many of the home-care needs can be met by nurses, the multidisciplinary team, involving social workers, attendants, physical therapists, and the volunteers, is essential if the AIDS patient is to remain home. These team members work closely with the primary physician to develop a plan of care that will sustain the person in the home environment. This multidisciplinary approach will help both the patient and the team members deal with the physical and psychological problems related to the diagnosis of AIDS and the terminal stages of the illness, including bereavement support.

Traditional home care does not concern itself that much with bereavement issues. The hospice care program emphasizes emotional support for the entire family, especially when dealing with death and dying. For the friends and family survivors of an AIDS death, the bereavement process is quite complicated. Skilled bereavement counselors will provide needed support and assistance to the lover, family, and friends of the deceased, even for a period after death has occurred. Zimmerman states that the purpose of hospice bereavement care is to provide comfort, understanding, support, and information to surviving relatives and friends in an effort to alleviate the distress of bereavement and promote the most favorable outcome possible.[37] As members of the hospice team, the social worker and nurse each need to make one or two bereavement follow-up visits. A bereavement volunteer should be assigned to provide ongoing support and counseling to the friends or family members.

NOTES

1. R. Buckingham, *Care of the Dying Child: A Practical Guide for Those Who Help Others* (New York: Continuum, 1990).

2. W. Bulkin and H. Lukashok, "Rx for Dying: The Case for Hospice," *New England Journal of Medicine* 318, no. 6 (1988): 316–78.

3. G. Friedland, "Clinical Care in the AIDS Epidemic," *Daedalus* 118 (1989): 67–78.

4. Bulkin and Lukashok, "Rx for Dying."

5. J. Schoefferman, "Care of the AIDS Patient," *Death Studies* 12 (1988): 446.

6. Bulkin and Lukashok, "Rx for Dying."

7. Friedland, "Clinical Care in the AIDS Epidemic."

8. C. Tsoukas, "The Dying Leper Syndrome," *Journal of Palliative Care* 4 (1988): 13–14.

9. U.S. Department of Health and Human Services, Centers for Disease Control, "Review of the CDC Surveillances Case Definition for Acquired Immunodeficiency Syndrome," *Morbidity and Mortality Weekly Report* (Supplement) 36, no. 1S (1987): 15.

10. L. Altman, "AIDS Tests of Health Care Workers Called Unnecessary," *New York Times*, 23 February 1991, p. 9.

11. Ibid.

12. U.S. Department of Health and Human Services, Centers for Disease Control, "Recommendations for Prevention of HIV Transmission in Health Care Settings," *Morbidity and Mortality Weekly Report* 36, no. 2S (1987): 15.

13. Institute of Medicine, *Confronting AIDS: Update 1988* (Washington, D.C.: National Academy Press, 1988).

14. Altman, "AIDS Tests."

15. Friedland, "Clinical Care in the AIDS Epidemic."

16. C. Clark et al., "Hospice Care: A Model for Caring for the Person with AIDS," *Nursing Clinics of North America* 23 (1988): 851–62.

17. V. Moss, "The Mildmay Approach," *Journal of Palliative Care* 4 (1988): 105.

18. W. Haseltine, "Prospects for the Medical Control of the AIDS Epidemic," *Daedalus* 118 (1989): 14.

19. H. Anderson and P. MacElveen-Hoehn, "Gay Clients with AIDS: New Challenges for Hospice Programs," *Hospice Journal* 4 (1988): 38–39.

20. J. O'Connor et al., "Does Care Exclude Cure in Palliative Care?" *Journal of Palliative Care* 2 (1986): 11–15.

21. P. Mansell, "AIDS: Home, Ambulatory, and Palliative Care," *Journal of Palliative Care* 4 (1988): 31–32.

22. Ibid.

23. S. Librach, "Who's in Control? What's in a Family?" *Journal of Palliative Care* 4, no. 1 (1988): 1–12.

24. V. Mor, *Hospice Care Systems: Structure, Process, Costs, and Outcome* (New York: Springer Publishing, 1987), pp. 140–76.

25. J. Durham and F. Cohen, *The Person with AIDS* (New York: Springer Publishing, 1987), pp. 21–37.

26. D. Abrams et al., "AIDS: Caring for the Dying Patient," *Patient Care* 23, no. 19 (1989): 23–36.

27. Ibid.

28. Clark et al., "Hospice Care."

29. Abrams, "AIDS: Caring for the Dying Patient."

30. Clark et al., "Hospice Care."

31. Ibid.

32. T. Stephany, AIDS and the Hospice Nurse," *Home Health Nurse* 8, no. 2 (1990): 141–54.

33. Clark et al., "Hospice Care."

34. J. Rhymes, "Hospice Care in America," *Journal of the American Medical Association* 264, no. 3 (1990): 369–72.

35. Bulkin and Lukashok, "Rx for Dying."

36. I. Corles and M. Pittman-Lindeman, *AIDS Principles, Practice and Politics* (New York: Hemisphere Publishing, 1989), pp. 58–72.

37. J. Zimmerman, *Hospice: Complete Care for the Terminally Ill* (Baltimore and Munich: Urban and Schwarzenberg, 1986), pp. 98–112.

8

Grief Management

The experience of loss and the expression of grief are common to all humanity, yet each culture has its own unique way of experiencing them. Not only each culture, but each person will experience grief in different way; no two experiences are exactly the same. Because grieving is such an important part of hospice, this chapter discusses different reactions to grief among different groups of people as well as issues associated with grieving. The following definitions are provided for clarification to the reader.

Bereavement: Bereavement is a state involving loss. In fact, to *bereave* means to take away from, to rob, to dispossess. The term usually implies that the loss produces unhappiness.

Grief: Grief refers to the feelings of anger, guilt, sorrow, and confusion that can arise when you have suffered a loss or are bereaved. It seems fair to say that you can't grieve without being bereaved, but you can be bereaved and not grieve. Although the process of grieving seems necessary for full recovery from a significant loss, grieving itself means pain and suffering.

Mourning: Mourning is the overt expression of grief and bereavement. The ways in which we mourn are heavily influenced by our culture; we may dress in black or white, attend funerals or say prayers at home, drink and laugh at the wake, or take tranquilizers and cry at the funeral.[1]

EXPRESSIONS OF GRIEF :

There is no "correct" way to express grief, but some expressions appear to lead to more effective recovery from the distressing aspects of experiencing the death of a loved one. Grief can be expressed physically, cognitively, affectively, or behaviorally. *Cognitively,* grief may take the form of disbelief, confusion, preoccupation with thoughts of the dead person and perhaps of the dying process, and encounters with the dead person in ways that make that person seem still alive. *Affective* ways to express grief may be depression, sadness, sorrow, relief, guilt, anger, or denial.[2]

  Physical expressions of grief may include the following:

- a hollow feeling in stomach
- a tight feeling in chest or throat
- oversensitive reactions to noise
- a sense of depersonalization (nothing seems real)
- breathlessness, feeling short of breath
- muscular weakness
- lack of energy
- dry mouth[3]

Behavioral expressions of grief may include the following:

- sleep disturbances, such as insomnia or sudden awakening
- appetite disturbances, usually undereating
- absent-minded behavior, such as getting lost while driving because of taking a wrong turn, or missing appointments.
- social withdrawal from other people, especially early in the mourning process
- dreams of the dead person, both normal dreams and nightmares
- sighing a great deal
- restless over-activity, such as having to get out of the house or not being able to concentrate on reading the newspaper

- crying

- avoiding reminders of the deceased

- visiting places or carrying objects that are reminders of the dead person (the opposite of avoiding these reminders)

- treasuring objects that belonged to the deceased,
such as keeping her room exactly as it had been,
including clothing in the closet[4]

LOSS IN CHILDHOOD

The death of a parent is potentially the most traumatic
experience that can occur in childhood. Because it is
such a shock, children go through a period of denial
until they can come to terms with reality. Even though
there is an intellectual understanding of what has occurred, until there is an emotional understanding, children will be unable to continue emotional and psychological growth. Knowing and understanding that a loved
person is dead is not the same as accepting it.

The knowledge that children have concerning the
death of the parent is extremely important to their psychological well-being. An easier adjustment can be
made if they are allowed to know what is happening
during the various stages of the parent's death. Children who are sheltered from the experience of death
somehow feel that they are to blame for the death or disappearance of their parent. This can have severe reper-
cussions later, emotionally or psychologically. Once

children have integrated the death, it will always be part of them, but they will be able to move on to new relationships, and have fond memories of the dead parent that won't overwhelm them. Successful resolution of the mourning process implies that the deceased will remain a "living memory" without the pain that originally accompanied the grief reaction.[5]

For years it was believed that children could not handle a traumatic event such as death. They were often told that the person who had died had "gone to sleep" or had gone on a long journey. Many of these children wondered why the individual had left without saying good-bye, and some felt that they had done something wrong to cause the person to leave so suddenly. Because of these conflicting feelings, the children would suffer from guilt, depression, and anger at having been abandoned. Feeling deserted, the children wonder what they may have done to cause the beloved one to leave. They recall angry feelings they had toward the deceased or their refusal to honor a request from that person. These children believe that their thoughts or actions might, in some way, be responsible for the disappearance of the loved one.

Today, parents and psychologists alike are realizing that children do have a concept of death, and when helped, they can integrate and adjust to the death of someone very close. Children are exposed to death every day of their lives. If they don't see it on television, then they see it when a cat catches a bird, or when they squash a bug.

When children learn of the death of a parent, their initial reaction is one of shock, disbelief, and denial.

190 The Handbook of Hospice Care

Death is hard for them to recognize. Youngsters usually experience feelings of ambivalence, unrecognized hostility, as well as conscious and unconscious anger directed at the dead parent. That person left and now they are abandoned. For some children, tears are the beginning of relief; in others repeated and prolonged inconsolable sobbing occurs with no sign of diminishing. Some children have such an intense sadness that it is hard for the remaining parent to console them.

With a parent's help, children can work through their grief. Parents should not be afraid to show emotion in front of their children. Instead of being harmful and upsetting, it can be helpful and comforting for the child to see that the parent is also suffering a loss. Seeing the parent composed may confuse children, and they may wonder how something that could make them hurt so much would not affect the parent. Some children might think there is something wrong with them. It offers great support in facing their own tears to see and feel a parent's ability to experience fully his own grief.[6]

To help them deal with their grief, children have several coping mechanisms, one of which is *withdrawal.* Customary activities or mementos may hold too much remembrance. As protection from being overwhelmed by sad feelings, some children will shy away from activities and objects that used to give them so much pleasure.

Denial is another grief reaction to the death of a parent. It is exhibited in the continuation of rituals in which the children and their deceased parent participated together. If children immediately return to play after being informed of the death, it should not be taken as an indication of callousness or lack of concern. It is just a form of denial. These actions are in reality a return to the familiar to allow young minds time to assimilate and accept what is horrible, new, and unfamiliar.[7]

Children should be able to work through grief at their own level of emotional and cognitive maturity. They should be encouraged to express their feelings, concerns, and questions, all of which should be answered with sympathy, candor, clarity, and an invitation to ask more questions. Most important is that children be told that death is real, irreversible, and no one's fault.

Remembrance and *longing* constitute another step in the bereavement process children experience. Attachment to a love object is never withdrawn easily. The unavailability of the loved person calls forth longing. Through this remembrance and longing process children are able to detach themselves from the dead parent.

Youngsters may show a certain amount of *ambivalence* and *hostility* toward the parent in his attempt to lessen the emotional impact that their memories have on them. Defense mechanisms can be the greatest interference in attempts by grieving children to accept the fact of death, and then to continue on with life.

Surviving parents who are aware of these defenses can help a child to overcome them. One means could be the act of helping the young person do something previously done with the dead parent, and acknowledging the fact that it does produce a sad feeling, but one that will diminish in time. When a surviving parent cannot mourn adequately or cannot empathize with the child's feelings of loss, the youngster sometimes experiences the barrier as a partial loss of the living parent.

If the parent dies of a long-term illness, it can have

either a beneficial or a harmful effect on the child's mourning process; the difference lies in what the youngster was told concerning the illness, and in the child's involvement with the parent during the illness. Under the right circumstances, contact with the dying can be useful to a youngster. It may diminish the mystery of death and help develop more realistic ways of coping. It can open avenues of communication that reduce the loneliness often felt by both the living and the dying. The opportunity to bring a moment of happiness to a dying individual may help a child feel useful.

A child taken to visit a parent in the hospital should be prepared for changes, especially if there have been drastic ones since the child last saw the parent; there should be warnings about any machinery that might be in the room. Instead of being told that the parent is going to die, which would put a strain on the time left together, the child should be informed that the doctors are doing all they can for the parent and they can't be sure about what will happen in the future. "The terminally ill patient should explain that she or he has no control over death, but that they are receiving the best care possible and will remain alive as long as possible."[8]

An honest approach to what is happening is best for children. Later problems can be avoided if youngsters are allowed to participate with the rest of the family in mourning, going to the funeral, and visiting the grave. Otherwise, the sudden removal of the loved one, without explanation or concrete evidence of the death, may induce in children the image that they somehow caused the parent to leave, a misconception that can result in lifelong guilt. This is also true if the lost one is a sibling.

Every child has had occasional angry thoughts about siblings, and if the reason for illness and death is not explained, the child may imagine his own anger to have been the cause.

If the parent or sibling dies in a hospice inpatient or home-care program, the surviving child will in all likelihood have fewer difficulties. Frequent visits, and participation in the dying person's care, help make the death more acceptable and leave the survivors with fewer regrets. It still may be difficult for the child to face the reality of loss, for even in the case of a prolonged illness the youngster may have entertained hopes of recovery.

When faced with the reality of their loss, some children are not able to express their feelings in socially acceptable ways, and explode in serious antisocial acts. Bottled-up distress over the death of a parent may manifest itself in resistance to normal cooperation, change in moods, minor physical symptoms such as aches and pains or inability to sleep or eat, as well as more serious symptoms, such as lying, stealing, and bed wetting.[9] Various behavioral patterns can be a warning that psychiatric help may be needed for a bereaved child. For example, the child who appears to show no grief at all may be in trouble and have problems much later in life. If a child maintains an unshakable fixation on the lost love object; if he continues to believe for more than a week or so that the dead person will return, he may need aid to give up his fantasy and deal with the reality of the situation. If the child ceases to function in school or turns to severe delinquent activities (some decline in school work is to be expected, but complete absorption in daydreams is a call for help), then intervention, such as counseling, is called for. The child whose anger leads him to strike out at society by stealing or other illegal and unsociable acts also needs help.[10]

Parents should recognize the fact that in order for children to mourn the dead parent, they need more than their own recollections of that parent; children also require the surviving parent's help in confirming the objective truth of memories, of both positive and negative aspects of the dead parent's personality. More facts about the dead parent are needed in each new stage of the child's personality development. In this way the parent is included in the children's growing personality, and yet the children can differentiate themselves from the parent.[11]

The ambivalence a child feels at a parent's death is also present if the deceased is a sibling. While mourning the lost brother or sister, the child may feel relief that the parents are no longer occupied with caring for the terminally ill sibling. A recurring theme among surviving siblings seems to be that the parents were so lost in their own grief at the time that they were unable to comfort the living children. These children may feel quite alone at this time and may wonder if they might become ill with the disease from which the sibling died. It is a good idea for parents, and deceased children's doctors, to reassure surviving siblings that they are well and unlikely to become ill with the same disease. If the disease was hereditary (such as cystic fibrosis) and a brother or sister does have it, it may help to point out that the disease is different in each case, and that new treatments are being discovered all the time.

Some hospices offer support groups for siblings of terminally ill or deceased children. Lacking them, the hospice will know of available resources in the community. A support group of other siblings in similar situations can help a child resolve feelings of loss and guilt.

In conclusion, we must remember that adults caring for a bereaved child must appreciate the limits of what can be done to alleviate the child's sadness. The surviving parent needs to accept and respect the youth's feelings. The primary task is to comfort and support children as they long for the return of their loved one, grapple to understand the permanence of the loss, and, in their unique way, experience the mourning process.

BEREAVED MOTHERS AND FATHERS

The loss of a child is one of the greatest sorrows an adult can face. Although both are parents with the same loss, we will discuss mothers and fathers separately, for in our culture men and women grieve differently and society expects different behavior from them during periods of mourning. Harriet Sarnoff Schiff described this experience very well in her book *The Bereaved Parent*. She was offered much sympathy after her son died and she was allowed to cry and mourn freely, while her husband was expected to suppress all outward signs of grief and to go to work as usual. Self-help groups for bereaved parents also reflect this, with mothers attending more frequently and expressing their grief more openly. Fathers are often asked, "How's your wife?" and rarely asked how they are bearing the loss themselves. It is beyond the scope of this chapter to discuss the reasons for this, or the history of mourning customs in our culture, but one can recall movies and novels in which women weep following a death while men remain silent or subdued.

Everyone grieves in his or her own way, and these variations sometimes place a great strain upon a marriage. If a marital relationship can sustain the death of a child, then the marriage is likely to be very stable. It is estimated that as many as 90 percent of bereaved couples have serious marital difficulties after their child's death.[12] One possible cause of this is that each parent is going through grief at a different pace and can seldom afford the psychological energy to support the other. This is another area where a hospice bereavement program can benefit many families. The death of a child is very different from the death of parents or siblings. For a woman, having a child is a unique event. The long period of pregnancy, delivery, and early nurturing builds special bonds that only a mother has with her child. To lose a child is like losing a part of herself, which indeed she has.

Mothers

The mourning process of a woman can last for months or even years. Some women mourn for a lifetime if proper intervention is not provided. Most women will go through a period of feeling dazed and depressed. They will feel numb, angry, guilty, and sometimes wish they were dead. There is a process of pining and thinking for a fleeting moment that the child is back. Sometimes the mother will actually forget and call the child, or even buy the child something.

Keep in mind that parents, and especially mothers, will grieve in many different ways depending upon the age of the child, the child's previous health, and the closeness of the relationship with the parent. It takes time for a woman to develop memories of her child.

The first stage of mourning, one of shock and disbelief, usually lasts a day or even longer. The numbness a woman feels is really a form of self-protection that allows her time to attend to immediate matters. If this state of shock and disbelief persists for several days, it is a sign that something is wrong, an indicator of unyielding grief. Other immediate effects of bereavement for the mother may be feelings of abandonment, rejection of the facts involving the death, accident proneness, self-blame, or vengefulness toward someone she blames for the death. Many times a mother will blame God or even her husband. Many women will doubt their adequacy as mother or wife.[13]

During the second stage, that of longing for the child, the mother will experience waves of memories and images of her child. Memories can be triggered by a toy, a holiday, or a playmate the child had in school. This preoccupation with the dead child is actually a gradual adaptation to the loss, and is part of the grief process. During this stage, which lasts for about a year, peaking at about three months, some of the following behavior may be observed: escaping from the death through drugs or alcohol, by moving to a new house, or through social distractions or work may occur; other occurrences may be removing all reminders of the child, deliberately forgetting or refusing to talk about the child,

The Handbook of Hospice Care

becoming a recluse, identifying with the child, reat-
taching affections to a new child to replace the deceased
one, or constantly espousing charities or causes usually
related to the child's illness.[14]

Most of these behavior patterns take time to develop.
Some women think they must fit into a model when
they are going through the bereavement process. They
feel guilty if they do not follow the standard pattern of
grief. But in our culture, there is no standard for death.

It is hard for a parent, especially a mother, to return
to the normal way of life. She wants to talk about the
loss, but her friends and family may be reluctant to listen. It is very important to let a woman express her
thoughts and feelings about her child's death. If she
keeps them bottled up inside, the grieving process will
take much longer. Talking about painful memories and
episodes of sadness will help the mother, and gradually
the past will become much easier to talk about. The
emptiness will remain for shorter periods and will go
away for longer periods. In this way the mother is saying good-bye, bit by bit, and the pain is not so harsh.
Soon, when the good-bye is complete, all the mother has
left are the memories of the child, and the pain has
gone. If the good-bye is never completed, the bereaved
mother will never return to the world of living or become
active and productive again.

Fathers

The great strain the death of a child places upon the father often goes unrelieved. Men in our society are ex-

pected to remain in control, even in times of crisis or emotional upheaval. Society's view of the traditional male role may be the basis for much misunderstanding of the grieving father. Of course, grief reactions differ from father to father, but generally, men display less emotion than women. Their denial of feelings may lead to increased use of alcohol or narcotics, severe depression, withdrawal from everyday activities, or other long-term traumatic conditions.

Interestingly, the anticipatory grief associated with the care of a terminally ill child may cause more emotional trauma for a father than for a mother. Mothers are traditionally the main caregivers, while fathers are breadwinners. If the child is in a care facility, the father may visit infrequently, thus failing to accommodate himself to the problems of the child, the mother, and the staff that he encounters. Fathers are more likely to react by withdrawing totally from the situation; they can easily resort to immersion in their work. Mothers will accept the inevitable first because they have seen more crises and welcome death as relief. It is no wonder that parents are rarely in the same stages of grief. As death approaches, some fathers cannot stay in the room. They feel helpless and useless, and they fear they will break down and lose control. The emotions that are voiced are tremendous guilt, frustration, anger, and self-hatred. Most fathers remain withdrawn and closed-mouthed. Mothers may resent this and say, "He doesn't care, he isn't grieving at all."

Sometimes it is easier for a father to talk to another bereaved father about the loss, someone who has been through the experience. In fact, both parents may find it easier to talk with others who have shared a similar experience, others who know how hard it is to go on with daily living, who understand how long it takes for the ache to subside. Bereavement support groups (organized in nearly every hospice) can help a husband and wife through the grieving process, with patience and understanding. Hospice bereavement programs can also make referrals for other kinds of counseling (when not offered at the hospice), such as financial advice for couples burdened with debts after a child's prolonged illness. Such burdens, when couples are already overwhelmed with grief, can be staggering. Indeed, bereavement support is essential for the survival of many families.

Family members need each other's compassion and love to recover from the loss of a child. Patience and gentleness can ease the pain of grief and allow the wounds to heal.

PARENTAL LOSS IN ADULTHOOD

Many hospice patients are older people suffering from a terminal illness who will leave grown children behind. Most adults do feel grief over the loss of a parent, including some shock and numbness. Many people observe change in their self-image following the death of a parent. For example, they begin to focus on what really is important in their lives. This sometimes alters their demeanor and actions toward the people with whom they interact. Others become aware of the emergence of a part of themselves that reflects the dead parent.

As with other sorts of bereavement, there is a tendency to idealize the lost parent. Sometimes there is a negative tendency as well (remembering the dead parent as worse than he or she probably was). Those who have the most difficulty with mourning and grief are those with unfinished business. When the survivor feels ambivalence toward the deceased, as well as some responsibility or guilt over the past, there may be more difficulty resolving the grief.

Daughters often have (or report) more difficulty with loss after the death of a parent. This may be because daughters tend to maintain closer ties with parents in adulthood, or because women feel less inhibited about expressing grief. Also, daughters are more likely to have attended to the parent during a terminal illness. When this occurs with hospice support, there may well be fewer problems, and less unfinished business.

Daughters and sons who cared for a parent with hospice support, either at home or at the inpatient unit, will have received much support and will have experienced a period of anticipatory grief. During the bereavement period they will receive visits from the hospice bereavement team. In addition, friends and family, religious and philosophical beliefs, and urgent life concerns can all help the adult child to cope. Most adults see the loss of their parent as painful, but experience some beneficial growth.

The meaning of the loss of a parent is often largely internal and symbolic. The death of a parent marks the end of one of our oldest relationships, and it will affect relationships with survivors.

WIDOWS AND WIDOWERS

It has been said that the loss of a child is the loss of the future; with the loss of a parent comes the loss of the past, but when the loss is that of a spouse, one seems to lose the present. Widowers and widows have so many adjustments to make that, again, the need for hospice bereavement programs is self-evident.

The psychological response to bereavement involves a period, often a year or two, of grief and mourning during which the survivor's ability to function is somewhat impaired. It does not generally involve pathological symptoms such as headache, loss of appetite, muscle spasms, or disturbed sleep unless previous symptoms were present. There is good evidence that the loss of a spouse may be followed by deterioration in physical and mental health of the survivor.[15] There appear to be increases in illness, accident, and mortality rates among spouses of the deceased, perhaps partially as a result of physical exhaustion, loneliness, and grief itself.[16] Middle-aged widows have been shown to experience almost universally certain emotional problems, among them depression, anxiety, apathy, insomnia, a sense of the presence of the deceased, and difficulty in accepting the fact of loss.[17]

A study of 109 widowed persons during the first month of their bereavement found that the most common symptoms were crying, depressed feelings, difficulty in sleeping, impaired concentration, poor memory, lack of appetite and weight loss, and heavy reliance on sleeping pills and tranquilizers.[18] During the process of bereavement, preoccupation with the image of the deceased partner and the quality of the feelings aroused by that image, to the exclusion of other experiences, usually diminishes as survivors accept their new role and begin reorganizing their lives. This change occurs to the extent that the widowed persons are able to adopt new modes of interaction, new pastimes and relationships.

It has been determined that preparation for the loss lessens the potential for abnormal or extreme grief reactions. The duration and the nature of the illness, particularly with respect to changes in the dying individual, also appear to influence the grief reaction of the survivor, thus affecting later readjustment. For example, if the patient displayed anger toward the loved one, the loved one may feel guilty and experience symptoms caused by patient-induced guilt. The widow who is allowed, by friends and by society, to express her thoughts and display her emotions is likely to have less difficulty working through the grief process and thus will begin her readjustment earlier. The greater the variety of socially valuable roles and functions from which the widow may choose, the more she is reoriented with a sense of meaning, purpose, and productivity in life, which are essential to her identity.

Change in economic status particularly burdens a surviving woman. Loss of income may result in financial insecurity, personal anxiety, and frustration. The widow may be forced to seek employment, but often she may lack adequate employable skills. Equally burdensome is the death of the spouse, usually the husband, who handled all the financial affairs. The survivor feels helpless and inept to cope with daily issues. The presence of training programs or employment counselors may make a large difference in the widow's adaptation.

The social situation of the widow at the time of and following the death of her spouse affects her readjustment. Particularly important is the availability of meaningful relationships, both similar to and different from the one cut off by the loss. The cultural patterns of the widow and her society, including rituals and religious beliefs, are significant in facilitating or inhibiting mourning.

Giving up the old role of wife and seeking a new identity is very difficult. The widow must manage many unaccustomed tasks that were formerly done by her husband. In other ways, also, it is difficult to find the way to a new identity. Diane Kennedy Pike described this experience and the transition from the dynamic relationship of a wife to feeling like a nonentity as a widow. When interviewed, or engaged to speak in public, she was invariably referred to as "the widow of James Pike" (a well-known author, speaker, and bishop), and found that people expected his views and not hers. As she says, "to be 'Jim's widow' felt restrictive, like having identity only in relation to what once was, to be wedded to the past."[19]

Most widows have considerable financial strain to which they must adjust. The medical bills may have exceeded insurance reimbursement during a long terminal illness. If the husband was the major wage earner, the widow may face a limited income and lowered standard of living. If there are children to raise as well, she has further considerations.

In our culture, the widow may very well be denied the support she needs. "Every widow discovers that people who were previously friendly and approachable become embarrassed and strained in her presence. Expressions of sympathy often have a hollow ring and offers of help or social interaction ("We'll have to get together. I'll call you") are not followed up. It often happens that only those who share the grief or themselves suffered a major loss remain at hand. It is as if the widow has become tainted with death in much the same way as the funeral director.[20] In some instances, widowed people also have problems with married friends who now see the widowed as competition for their spouses. This perceived threat further reduces the amount of support the widow receives from society.

As a whole, American cultural patterns do not indicate a tolerance for expressions of bereavement. Geraldine Palmer described her own experience of bereavement as follows: "Not only did people not want to talk about my husband's death, they couldn't feel or understand my pain, my bewilderment, my abject grief. Not my parents, my brother, my friends, relatives, nor psychiatrist."[21]

Emmy Gut states that the middle-aged woman who loses her husband by death is likely to feel intense preoccupation with her own physical health, and to be plagued with fears of being physically or emotionally alone in the face of terminal illness and death.[22] Unless the widow is encouraged to express her feelings, her fears may be repressed without being resolved, thus enhancing risks for mental and physical breakdown. Talking about her loss helps the widow accept it.

While widows have recently earned a place in society's attention, widowers, a somewhat rarer and quieter species, are often ignored. There is a tendency to assume that the widower must be getting along all right because we do not hear much from or about him. In fact, studies of recently widowed men demonstrate an increase in mortality, an increased tendency toward depression, general symptoms of disturbance in sleep, appetite, and weight, greater consumption of alcohol and tranquilizers, a tendency to need and seek help for emotional problems, difficulty in making decisions, and an augmentation of acute physical symptoms. Two separate studies have established a significant correlation between the widower's early stage of bereavement and an increase in widower mortality. One recorded an increase in the death rate among 4,486 widowers of almost 40 percent during the first six months of bereavement.[23]

The widower's responses to bereavement can be traced in relationship to important events in the bereavement process. Newly bereaved widowers responded to the impact of death with shock, anguish, and numbness. They were apt to report a feeling of "dismemberment"; feeling "like both my arms were being cut off." Widowers were apt to feel "choked up" but most resisted the urge to cry or make a scene. Pangs of grief or episodes of severe anxiety and psychological pain during which the widower strongly missed his spouse began within a few hours after the impact of bereavement and usually reached a peak during the second week. Feelings of panic, a dry mouth, and other autonomic activity were also pronounced. Deep sighing respiration, restless but aimless hyperactivity, and difficulty in concentrating on anything but thoughts of loss were common.[24]

Typically, the widower was control- and reality-oriented. He was unlikely to speak openly about his feelings. He did not seek out opportunities to share either the events related to his loss or his personal reactions to it. He was likely to feel uncomfortable with direct emotional expression and attempted to maintain control of his feelings, as it was considered a weakness to let go.

Widowers indicated that most felt friends and family expected them to be strong, to hold up and not break down. One widower said that he had succeeded in suppressing his own feelings until he saw his father weeping at the funeral. After reacting to his father's outburst with shocked surprise, he realized that crying was an acceptable thing to do at a funeral. He himself also started to cry.

Some widowers expressed surprise and fear at the intensity of their emotions and imaginings after the impact of bereavement. They feared going mad when strong feelings of anger overcame them. Many reported vivid nightmares, distractibility, and difficulty in remembering everyday matters. Some expressed concern over how they would be able to manage in the months to come. Many experienced guilt feelings and were likely to blame themselves for what they did or did not do in relation to the death: "I wasn't sensitive enough to her" or "I should have made things easier."

Widowers are typically intolerant of their impulse to dwell upon the past and forced themselves to focus on the immediate realities of their situation. They resume work roles and other functions within a short period of time after their spouse's death. Pangs of grief become less frequent and occur usually only when triggered by a particular memento or event.

When the adjustment of widows and widowers was compared, researchers at first reported that widowers overall seemed more adjusted to their loss. The men showed less overt distress after bereavement than the women and appeared to have a much better psychological and social adjustment a year later. They had returned to work roles and previous functions sooner than the widows, and they began to date earlier.

However, a close look at the quality of the widowers' lives, including the occupational sphere, indicated a significant decrease in energy, competence, and satisfaction. At follow-up, two to four years after the death of the spouse, it was the men who were found to have taken longer to recover. Even though the widower appeared more adjusted, it did not mean that he had worked through his attachment to his late wife or the feelings stirred up since her death.

HOSPICE BEREAVEMENT PROGRAMS

As has been discussed previously, bereavement follow-up is a necessary component of the hospice philosophy. The number and intensity of the adjustments families must make to the loss of a loved one clearly demonstrates the need for ongoing care for the survivors. The hospice concept of including the family in the unit of care is practical socially, as bereavement programs can help reduce the unhealthy behaviors which may arise from grief (e.g., delinquency, divorce, and drug or alcohol abuse).

Hospice helps families prepare for bereavement as well. Volunteers help patients and families prepare wills, discuss funerals, and plan for the future. Together the patient and family prepare themselves for the inevitable. They are able to discuss their feelings and deal with any unresolved business. All those involved are able to come to terms with the death, and survivors are likely to have fewer (if any) feelings of guilt about how the relationship with their loved one ended.

The greatest grief may occur weeks or months after the death. Immediately following the death, family and friends give much support. The funeral service itself may also focus community support on the newly bereaved. However, after the funeral, most friends and relatives go back to their own lives, hopeful that the bereaved will recover quickly and with little help. It is during this time that bereavement brings great loneliness, and often the unresolved need to talk about the loved one and the experience of death.

Hospice bereavement programs, which customarily make no charge for their services, usually begin with a visit to the family one month after the death. The bereavement team includes a counselor or nurse and a highly trained volunteer. Usually the volunteer and the hospice home-care nurse have helped with funeral planning and attended the funeral, so the family has often had previous contact with some member of the bereavement team. The team also includes the chaplain, the social worker, students, and volunteers. Assessments are made which take into consideration the welfare of the family and social adjustments that may arise after the loved one dies. Additional visits and outside help may be sought for those families that are not coping well. Visits continue, with assessment at three, six, and nine months. The needs of individual families vary, so not every family will require frequent visits. Another assessment visit is made at thirteen months, rather than at twelve months, since the anniversary of the death is a painful time for most. Assessment can add to a family's stress, and it may be inaccurate during a difficult time, such as at the anniversary of the death. Families are not forgotten and receive help from volunteers and the bereavement counselor. The anniversary is likely to be remembered in the support-group meeting for bereaved families, or in some other special way. Some families will be followed for up to two years, but for many the deepest grief will be over after the first year.

Hospice bereavement programs may include individual counseling, as well as the volunteers' visits, support groups, seminars on grief, and programs during the holidays. This last is particularly important, because holidays trigger memories of family gatherings and are often sad rather than happy times for the bereaved.

Risk factors in family members are noted during the initial bereavement visit. Such things as difficulty expressing feelings, family discord, dependency, clinically depressed moods, weight disturbance, or any other dysfunction may occur and are noted. The mourner's past history of losses is important also, as well as any present feelings of anger, guilt, or denial. The social supports of the family are assessed, as well as any chronic physical conditions. An adolescent, or a young woman with chil-

dren at home may have more difficulties that may require attention. Strengths might be social supports, a
sense of spirituality, enjoyable work, willingness to seek
help, and a good coping history with previous losses.

In the St. Mary's Hospice program in Tucson, Arizona, a home visit is made for assessment by a hospice
professional at one month with telephone visits occur-
ring until the home visit at thirteen months. Volunteers
supplement these with additional home visits and note
any problems that may require professional help. In addition, a support group meets once a week. Referrals are
made to other groups, depending upon the needs of the
bereaved. The program in Tucson also gives many seminars for bereaved families, with such topics as grief
and loss or stress reduction. Families are asked to fill
out questionnaires on features of the program they've
found most helpful, as well as any other suggestions for
helping others to cope with loss.

There are special programs throughout the year, and
the Christmas program seems especially beneficial as
well as being lovely. Bereaved family members, children,
friends, hospice staff, and volunteers receive a warm invitation to a Christmas pot-luck dinner. The program includes a candlelight service conducted by the hospice
chaplain. Following dinner (during which care is provided
for children) is an informal sharing of holiday experiences. Along with the invitation is sent a tactfully worded
questionnaire that asks if the family has been through a
holiday season since the death, what plans the family has
for the holiday, and ideas that might help others facing
the holidays after bereavement are solicited. These ideas
are shared after dinner and provide mutual benefit. Un-

fortunately, not all hospices have a program for the bereaved during holidays. Holidays, particularly Christmas, are a trying time when a family member is missing.

Counseling in the St. Mary's program is not limited to families whose loved one died of a terminal illness with hospice care. Referrals come from all over the city for those who need bereavement counseling, whether their loved one has been murdered, died during an accident, or committed suicide. Since there is little follow-up for those who suffer the shock of a sudden death, the hospice bereavement program is truly needed by the community. St. Mary's Hospice also does a good deal to educate the community on loss and grief, and some of the counselors help with other groups throughout town, such as Parents Who've Lost Children and a siblings group. These services include hospice bereavement counselors, but do not always take place in the hospice. They are open to all who have suffered these losses, not just the relatives of the terminally ill.

CONCLUSION

We all face many occurrences of grief and loss throughout our lives when events do not turn out as we would like them to. The most powerful and disrupting grief occurs after the death of a loved one and the effects are profound. Grief and loss affect so many people other than the bereaved (society as well as the family suffers when divorce, or poor mental and physical health follow a death) that a good hospice bereavement program not only is compassionate but is preventive medicine. Every one of us will be affected during our lives by a loss through death, and it makes sense to fund hospice bereavement programs as a community service. The hospice in Tucson is responding to the community's need for bereavement counseling, as well as education in dealing with grief, loss, and resultant stress. Families who have been through a terminal illness and death certainly need this service, but so do families who have had a sudden or violent loss. Families faced with medical expenses after a long illness are not likely to have the means to pay for bereavement follow-up. Since clearly the whole community benefits from a hospice bereavement program (especially when clients are not limited to hospice families), perhaps funds will come from the community for this. Perhaps someday death education, bereavement follow-up, and hospice bereavement programs will become the standard rather than the exception. Grief cannot be eliminated from life any more than death can, but it can be softened and resolved with compassionate, knowledgeable care.

NOTES

1. All definitions can be found in R. Kalish, *Death, Grief, and Caring Relationships* (Pacific Grove, Calif.: Brooks, Cole Publishing, 1981).
2. Ibid.
3. J. Worden, *Grief Counseling and Grief Therapy* (New York: Springer Publishing, 1981).
4. Ibid.
5. M. Shoor and M. Speed, "Delinquency as a Man-

214 The Handbook of Hospice Care

ifestation of the Mourning Process," *Psychiatric Quarterly* 37 (1963): 37.

6. E. Furman, *A Child's Parent Dies* (New Haven, Conn.: Yale University Press, 1974).

8. D. Dunton, "The Child's Concept of Death," in *Loss and Grief, Psychological Management in Medical Practice*, ed. B. Schoenberg (New York: Columbia University Press, 1970).

9. D. Hendin, *Death as a Fact of Life* (New York: Norton, 1973).

11. Furman, *A Child's Parent Dies.*

12. H. Schiff, *The Bereaved Parent* (New York: Penguin Books, 1978), p. 84.

13. C. Hollingsworth and R. Pasnau, *The Family in Mourning: A Guide for Health Professionals* (New York: Grune & Stratton, 1977).

14. E. Grollman, *Concerning Death: A Practical Guide for the Living* (Boston: Beacon Press, 1974).

15. C. Parkes, "Recent Bereavement as a Cause of Mental Illness," *British Journal of Psychiatry* 110 (1964): 198–204.

16. D. Kimmel, *Adulthood and Aging* (New York: Wiley, 1974), p. 433.

17. C. Parkes, *Bereavement: Studies of Grief in Adult Life* (New York: International University Free Press, 1972).

18. P. Clayton, J. Halikes, and W. Maurice, "The Bereavement of the Widowed," *Diseases of the Nervous System* 32 (1971): 597–604.

19. D. K. Pike, *Life Is Victorious: How to Grow Through Grief* (New York: Simon & Schuster, 1976).

20. Parkes, *Bereavement.*

21. G. Palmer, "Singles World," in *Alone and Surviving,* ed. R. Lindsay (New York: Walker, 1977).

22. Emmy Gut, "Some Aspects of Adult Mourning," *Omega* 5 (1974): 335.

23. B. Benjamin, M. Young, and C. Wallis, "Mortality of Widowers," *Lancet* 2 (1963): 454–56.

24. Parkes, *Bereavement.*

9

Hospice in Your Community

When looking for hospice care near your community, first call the National Hospice Organization (NHO) in Washington, D.C., for an updated listing of hospice programs near your home.* Make sure that all the philosophies of care as discussed earlier are practiced by your local hospice. A good hospice will have a coordinated home-care program with inpatient beds under a central autonomous hospice administration, have the means to control symptoms (physical, sociopsychological, and spiritual). It should have physician-directed services, provision of an interdisciplinary team, twenty-four-hours-a-day and seven-days-a-week services. The unit

---

*Information and a phone number for the NHO, as well as a listing of contacts for each state, are included in the appendix.

of care needs to include both the patient and family. Bereavement follow up programs should be available and the use of volunteers should be an integral part of the interdisciplinary team. The following is a list of components integral to a hospice.

COMPONENTS OF A HOSPICE

The Hospice Program: Home care should be the heart of the program, with coordinated inpatient backup if necessary. The program should also be autonomous, with freedom to make decisions regardless of whether or not the program is independent or housed within an acute-care facility.

Primary unit of care: Patient and family.

Symptom control: The hospice staff should be knowledgeable about the medical control of all physical symptoms. There should be attention also to the patient's nonphysical needs (emotional, social, and spiritual).

Medical director: A physician with a sound professional background should be the medical director. A group of well-meaning people alone cannot make a hospice.

Multidisciplinary team: Hospice services should be coordinated by a multidisciplinary team including a social worker, physical and occupational therapist, pastoral care provider, and consultant services as needed. The family and volunteers are also part of the team.

Volunteers: Trained selected volunteers help the hospice provide a wider variety of services.

Services available on call: Hospice services must be available seven days a week, twenty-four hours a day.

Bereavement follow-up: Depending upon the needs of the individual family, these services will vary, but they should be available.

Hospice education: Ideally, hospices have education programs available to the community.

Services based on need: Hospice services should be based on need rather than ability to pay.

When looking at an inpatient hospice (one in which patients can stay at the hospice and receive care), note the interaction between patients and staff (smiles, relaxed manner, personal interest and concern, etc.), the general atmosphere (cheerful, noninstitutional-looking), and the provisions for families and children. Can families stay overnight if they wish? Can relatives cook a special meal? Is there a place for children to play? Are there open (unrestricted) visiting hours?

If you or someone in your family needs a hospice, then you are on a very special journey together, and you will want a hospice that lives up to all the ideals described in this book.

HOSPICE AND THE COMMUNITY

Hospices throughout this country and in England have begun as local community efforts. Small groups of people, namely medical professionals, clergy, and concerned citizens, begin to meet, do research, and plan a hospice in their community. Next, a small grant or donation makes it possible to hire a staff member or to rent a small office (as in The Connecticut Hospice, Inc., in Branford). Sometimes the hospice begins as an office in someone's home (as in Hospice Orlando), able to offer a home-care program because of the volunteer efforts of a physician and nurses. Community support increases as friends and neighbors of patients hear about a patient's relief from pain and distress, and some give donations in gratitude or become volunteers. Hospice has truly been a grassroots movement of loving service with the community.

Individual hospices have had small community beginnings but each hospice has had to establish relations with the larger community. The public needs information about hospice, about what a hospice does and can do, and about the attitudes toward life and death that make the hospice concept work. Attitudes are changing, but a community may need additional help, or society's general denial of death may lead to prejudice against the hospice concept. When a small and carefully organized group in New Haven, Connecticut, began to search for a site for The Connecticut Hospice, Inc., community opposition in one town blocked settlement. The Connecticut Hospice, Inc. had to spend time preparing the community and educating possible neighbors before a site in Branford was agreed upon.

EVALUATION OF HOSPICE PROGRAMS

Further evaluations of hospice home care programs are necessary, as are evaluations of terminal care, which has been insufficiently assessed. Hospice program evaluation is essential to provide the rationale for decision making, to clarify the direction of future programming, and to supply the incentive to institute needed corrective measures. Appraisal of the degree to which programs meet the goals they were established and contracted to achieve is a necessary prerequisite for the extension of the hospice concept throughout the country.

Pressure for greater accountability will be placed upon hospice as it moves into the sphere of broad-range, nationwide, community service. The faith of the public it is to serve is fundamental to the program's universal acceptance. Evaluations of both home-care and inpatient hospice programs will help create the yardsticks by which one may measure standards of success, so that criteria may be validated and new criteria of effectiveness developed. Knowledge of the usefulness of specific procedures or techniques may help to identify logical applications of further efforts; advancing knowledge will affect assumptions, goals, and activities. In directing the course of future efforts in the field of terminal care, evaluations of the effectiveness of hospice care can increase the efficacy of innovative programs, point out areas requiring further research, and suggest possible alternatives to be explored. In the light of research findings, more desirable means for attaining the designated objectives may be proposed. It is vital to determine whether and how well hospice objectives are being met, and to ascertain the causes of specific successes or failures.

Evaluation studies and standards of care may help with reimbursement of a greater variety of hospice services. Now that the government has acknowledged the value and cost efficiency of hospice programs more funding may become available. Funding is especially needed for home-care programs and for extended care for the terminally ill in every age bracket. Though home and hospice care is considerably less expensive than standard acute care in hospitals, some families may suffer financially when insurance companies reimburse only aggressive treatment. Perhaps insurance companies will offer their policyholders more options to cover these realities in the future. I hope that both public and private funding and reimbursement will help families care for their relative at home if they wish, and will help inpatient hospice units to realize the highest ideals of care.

UNCOVERING THE HIDDEN ISSUE OF DEATH

Ongoing public education about the doings of a local hospice increases community awareness. There have been many programs on television during the past few years that have increased public attention to the needs of the dying and the bereaved. Numerous books, magazine articles, and public lectures have also helped to sensitize people to the needs of the terminally ill. We have come a long way since Elisabeth Kübler-Ross began the patient interviews that became *On Death and Dying,* and have come to talk more about death, but we still have a long way to go toward accepting death as a part of life. Visible hospices, or home-care hospice programs, help people see and accept that death is an inevitable part of life and should not be hidden away.

In the recent past (and even today), patients have

been sent to the hospital just because they were dying, even if the hospital had nothing to offer them. We tend to isolate and ignore that which frightens us, and we have been afraid of death. When home care takes place, neither the patient nor the family is isolated from the rest of the community, and death becomes a more naturally accepted event. In the hospice environment just as we do not deny death, we do not deny the grief of the bereaved.

Hospice can contribute to public awareness and acceptance by continuing to be a community within the community. Adults who have contact with a hospice may have a deeper understanding of the dying and of death, and they may see their own lives differently. Children also need such exposure, and may be taught from an early age that death is an expected and natural occurrence. The daycare centers on the grounds of St. Christopher's in London and The Connecticut Hospice, Inc., in Branford exist for the hospice staff and the children and grandchildren of the patients. These children bring vitality to hospice, and a sense of community with all the stages and ages of life, and in turn these children are given the gifts of compassion and learn that neither the old nor the terminally ill are frightening or foreign, but are simply their loving friends, grandparents, or parents at the end of life. These interactions strengthen community awareness, acceptance, and extend the hospitality of the hospice to all who enter the doors.

INTERAGENCY COOPERATION

As a part of the local community, hospice works with all other service groups in the area. Local groups may trade referrals and services and work together cooperatively. Visiting nurse associations can provide much support and many services to bed-ridden patients at home. Visiting nurses are usually available only during the day, Monday through Friday. Most hospice services are available twenty-four hours a day and on weekends. These two agencies can work together very harmoniously for mutual benefits. Hospice planners must understand local needs and know which human-service agencies are available in their area.

Working cooperatively with other agencies, and with the patient's personal physician, a hospice can reduce some of the fragmentation of medical services that plague many patients. Because each area of medical specialty works independently and there is no overall coordinator of health care, a patient and family may be sent from one doctor to another, from the intensive care unit to the coronary care unit or the oncology unit, and perhaps to the hospice unit. Fragmentation of services confuses, disturbs, and needlessly harasses the patient, and it is very expensive. This is the opposite of the caring community that is hospice, with its variety of skilled professionals who are part of one team. Because hospice care is so different in concept and practice from care the patient receives elsewhere, we must be careful not to let hospice become just another specialty, but we must integrate hospice services with the rest of the community.

It is hoped that hospice care will become standard care in the years to come and the hospice philosophy will be espoused by all health care personnel. Hospitality need not be only for the dying but, as in medieval times, for the woman in labor or the very ill as well. Most of the concepts of hospice work could very well apply to other health care agencies. Examples include the multidisciplinary team which sees to the needs of the family as well as the patient, or personal care which includes knowing the patients' names as well as their respective conditions. Also, relieving symptoms as well as seeking cures should be pursued with an attitude that views human beings as worthy of loving care, an attitude that accepts death as a natural occurrence. Concern and care can go very well with expert professional skills, and they do in hospice. I sincerely hope, too, that the education of medical and nursing students everywhere will include hospice's concepts of care and its philosophy of humane treatment of the dying and their families.

Within hospice, prevention of fragmentation is achieved through the variety of skills and social services offered. Counseling is available for patients and for families if needed; financial planning and help with making out a will are also available. Volunteers help the home-care patient with transportation, homemaking, caring for children, and performing various other services. Physicians, nurses, and therapists notice the patient's changing condition and prevent difficulties wherever possible. The patient's social and spiritual needs are given attention as well. Less urgent needs are also considered: some hospices have beauty salon equipment and have found volunteers with knowledge of body mas-

226 The Handbook of Hospice Care

sage and other skills. All these skilled people work together, not only as a team, but as a community.

REGULATION

Regulation is an essential factor in any skilled profession. The hospice medical staff must be expert in their science and have thorough knowledge of the newer methods of pain and symptom control. Particular emphasis is placed on the art of medicine, but the craft is essential, too. Pharmacologists must be knowledgeable and competent. Besides sympathy and friendly communication and teaching, the nurses give highly skilled care. A group of well-meaning people without these skills cannot make up a hospice. There must be uniform standards of care before the name "hospice" can be used. As Sandol Stoddard in his ground-breaking book on hospice care says: "Groups or individuals promising to provide 'an easy death' by removing the patient from medical professionals and performing some sort of hocus-pocus with or without the use of drugs are so far from being hospices that it is hard to imagine them trying to use the name. But there are reasons to believe that some will, and they should be guarded against."[1]

Hospice is becoming a popular idea which may tempt some to imitate superficial features of the concept without providing actual hospice care. I feel strongly that this would weaken the whole hospice movement and damage its credibility with the public as well as with possible sources of reimbursement. Agencies using the name without the meaning behind it would hurt the very people hospice is most concerned about: the patient and the family. Patients and families need information about hospice standards of care and what services they may expect. Further evaluations of present hospices can establish these standards and provide models for future hospices.

NOTE

1. Sandol Stoddard, *The Hospice Movement* (New York: Stein & Day, 1978).

10

The Future of Hospice Care

We have already discussed current hospice issues in chapter 3 and most of those issues focused on how to make hospice more available to children, people with AIDS, people living in rural areas, ethnically diverse cultures, and veterans. Some suggestions for accomplishing these goals were also offered. This chapter also focuses on issues, but looks at what's ahead for the future of hospice. It's important to look at these issues now, because they cannot be saved for the future; we need to be aware of them today in order to confront hospice issues with ease in the future. Topics which were listed in chapter 3 may also be included here if they are issues that need to be addressed both as current concerns and future ones.

EDUCATION

In our society death is viewed as a failure, a catastrophe, or an unnatural or immoral act from which we should be shielded. This attitude is an expected response to our medical technological "progress." The dying process can now be unnecessarily extended; it is increasingly mechanical and fearfully dehumanizing. But instead of working to combat such fears through education, most physicians tend to reinforce and promote them by refusing to accept the fact that there is a time to die. The hospice philosophy is slowly accepted in a society that refuses to acknowledge death as a natural and peaceful experience.

Education is one way of confronting our fear of death. Changing attitudes can be a long and drawn out process, but one of the most effective means to obtaining an acceptance of the hospice philosophy is through education, which can be presented in many different forms, ranging from teaching a volunteer how to be a good listener for patients to conducting an extensive research project.

Physicians

Physicians need to continue education in home health care, especially in the area of pain control. Current pain control methods need to continuously be improved for the benefit of the patient, his family, and again, a commitment to the hospice philosophy.

More research projects need to be undertaken in the area of hospice care in order to improve hospice care services. Incentives should be given to promote such research, and professional conferences need to be held regularly in order to exchange findings. Workshops, symposiums, publishing more health care journals, offering incentives for medical students to chose hospice care as a career are all ways of offering education to our physicians. Physicians will play a vital role in the continuing growth of hospice as a professional health care system.

Nursing, Medical, and Social Work Students

An important population to address, if not the most important population, is our future hospice workers. Currently, there are 126 medical schools and only two of them require hospice education courses or "practicing care of the dying" courses. Without classes available to teach about hospice care, the number of future hospice workers will be limited. We also need to train more "hospice researchers" to promote current and accurate data in hospice care. Classes in the curriculum should also require students to learn skills necessary to carry out complex home health care models of research.

More medical schools need to address hospice and care of the dying as an important part of the curriculum. These classes need to be a required part of the curriculum, which should also include the opportunity to have a credited internship under a hospice program. The opportunity for paid internships in home health-care positions should equal hospital positions. Currently this is not an option in medical schools.

Because of the AIDS epidemic, students need to be trained to deal on both a physical and a social level with patients who are infected with AIDS. Caring for people with AIDS is a consideration that will only become more and more of a reality in the future.

Better Management Training for Hospice CEOs

Most hospice chief executive officers come from a care-giver background. I am suggesting that CEOs of hospice have graduate training in management of health-care organizations (an M.B.A.) in combination with experience managing a complex organization.

Hospice is a sophisticated organization that needs a person with up-to-date health-care management skills. Some of these skills could include publicity, cost containment, public information, reimbursement mechanisms, and many more. These are skills that need to be in the hands of someone who has had formal and practical training in the area of home care management.

Nutrition

One area to which the hospice movement has not done justice is the arena of nutrition and hydration with respect to the terminally ill. We must understand the issues of nutrition and hydration as they affect our patients and their families.

Nutrition and hydration issues are of such importance for our terminally ill that I strongly recommend that a registered dietitian (R.D.) be made part of the hospice team. Based on educational experience, the R.D. is the individual most qualified to recommend to the hospice team the appropriate development of a nutritional plan for patients and family members who, under strain, may need counseling at this trying time of life.

Anorexia is a common problem with hospice patients. There are many interventions that can help with the problem associated with the loss of appetite and ensuing weight loss. The registered dietitian is the person who can provide advice and help in setting policies for each individual hospice patient.

There comes a time in the management of the terminally ill patient that certain nutritional policies change. The withholding of nutritional support from patients is one of the most controversial issues in medical circles today. Withholding nutritional support from a consenting patient is at times advisable and reasonable; it is nonetheless necessary to have experts like the R.D. to defend the decision.

The goals of hospice care should be approached from the physical, psychological, social, and spiritual needs and wishes of each individual patient and family. The extremes of patient control of foods and liquids, from being force-fed to withholding food and water, is of real concern for many. It is important to have the advice of an R.D. so the patient and family have the most accurate information possible on which to base their treatment decisions.

234 The Handbook of Hospice Care

EMPHASIZE HOME CARE,
NOT INPATIENT FACILITIES

Since the humble beginnings of the first American hospice home-care program in New Haven in 1974, hospices have been established in many communities throughout the country, and many more are in various stages of development. Hospice is a popular idea, and those who are involved in the movement are pleased to see its acceptance. It is encouraging to see how many hospices have been developed under the leadership of physicians and nurses who are changing traditional medical practice. However, overpopularity has its dangers. Hospice concepts are endorsed by both conservative and liberal politicians, by both young and old, and this is as it should be; but could hospice become a cliché like motherhood and apple pie, receiving sentimental endorsement without much thought for the underlying philosophy? Popularity can also lead to too many institutional hospices and not enough home care hospices.

If we ask the simple question, "where do we want to die?" I think most people would prefer to die at home. The thought of hospice is becoming associated with "building" a hospice. Hospice home-care programs can exist without an institution. We must not obscure our vision of hospice with buildings, or develop an "edifice" complex. Inpatient units are helpful as backup for the home-care program, and offer an alternative for some patients, but a hospice program can begin without a building. Hospice is an attitude toward life and toward death; it is an attitude of caring, of personal treatment that values the human spirit and sees each human being as worthy of love and care, regardless of age or physical condition. Hospice sees the patient as both giver and receiver. Hospice is more than a building, although buildings help facilitate hospice services. Hospice is a philosophy and practice of care.

REIMBURSEMENT

With the expansion of technology, more services can be provided in the home. Services such as parenteral and enteral nutrition (feeding intravenously as opposed to through the stomach), chemotherapy, and care of ventilator/trachdependent patients can now be provided in the home.[1] This reduces the need for more expensive hospitalization, but these services are costly for hospice to provide. Using more technology in the home also requires staff with additional training and may require longer visits. In order to bring technology into patients' homes, reimbursement agencies need to adjust for more time, more training, and more intense services.

INTERNATIONAL DEVELOPMENT OF HOSPICE PROGRAMS

Hospice care has become popular in the United States and it is continuing to grow. Currently, hospices exist in England, Germany, France, Costa Rica, Austria, Cuba, Canada, and most European countries. It's time to look further into the global community to spread the hospice concept. Hospice was originally developed in England and has continued to flourish in Europe, but the concept remains contained in the Eurocentric world. Even in the United States, only 15 percent of hospice patients are of non-European cultural descent.

With the spread of AIDS through Africa and Southeast Asia, it seems apparent that these areas could benefit from the hospice program. I would like to suggest the development of hospice in these non-European countries. The development can be funded by either government moneys or they could be supported by humanitarian organizations.

I have proposed a binational hospice to be developed along the Nogales, Mexico border. Careful bicultural considerations need to be made in order for the success of such a program. I look forward to the expansion of hospice for Mexican and American citizens who live along the border.

NOTE

1. National Association for Home Care, "NAHC 1995 Legislative Reports," *Blueprints for Action* (February 1995): 9–69.

Closing Thoughts

I hope that this handbook guides those who are curious, those about to make a decision regarding a loved one, and those who are beginning a career in the medical profession. This book was not intended to document all the research studies on death and dying, rather its purpose is just as the title says: a handbook. This book contains important information for those becoming new hospice volunteers!

The hospice approach centers on helping the dying and their loved ones to maintain the dignity and humanness of the dying process while providing sophisticated medical and nursing care. The focus of the hospice approach and philosophy is to help the dying to live as fully as possible during the time that remains. This entire book is built on the hospice philosophy which is necessary in order to understand the individual components of hospice care such as cost and administration.

I want the reader to feel comfortable with the concept of hospice care when they are through reading this handbook. This entails becoming familiar with the philosophy, history, administrative structure, and cost of hospice care. I especially want the reader about to make a decision about a terminally ill loved one to feel comfortable approaching hospice to help them encounter the trials and triumphs of the process of dying.

Good luck and God speed.

Appendix

National Hospice Organization
1901 North Moore Street, Suite 901
Arlington, VA 22209
(703) 243–5900
Fax (703) 525–5762
Hospice Helpline (800) 658–8898

The National Hospice Organization (NHO) was founded in 1978 as a nonprofit, public benefit, charitable organization advocating for the needs of terminally ill persons in America. NHO is the only national, nonprofit, membership organization devoted exclusively to the promotion of hospice care. NHO's members include more than 2,100 hospice programs, 48 state hospice organizations (plus the District of Columbia), and 3,900 hospice professionals.

Hospice is a comprehensive, medically supervised form of care which seeks to treat and comfort terminally ill patients and their families at home or in a homelike setting. NHO estimates that 340,000 patients and their families were served by hospice in the United States in 1994. Over the past five years, annual growth in the number of patients cared for by hospice nationwide has averaged 16 percent.

NHO provides a broad range of services to the public and its members. By calling the toll-free Hospice Helpline at (800) 658–8898, the public has access to information about the hospices in their community and hospice care in general. As a resource serving its members, NHO offers a wide variety of educational programs, technical assistance, and training curriculums. NHO also strives to influence health programs and public policies relative to hospice care and the needs of terminally ill persons and their families.*

Individual State Hospice Organizations

For information regarding the availability of hospice care in your state, call the Hospice Helpline at the toll-free number lised above, or contact the appropriate hospice listed below. Please note that the addresses and phone numbers for the state hospices are subject to change. In the event you are unable to reach the state organization you seek, please call the Helpline number, which will remain constant.

---

*This information has been supplied by NHO.

Alabama
Alabama Hospice Organization
2421 President's Dr., Ste. B–10
P.O. Box 231382
Montgomery, AL 36123–1382
(334) 213–7944 Fax (334) 213–7934

Alaska
Hospice of Alaska
3605 Arctic Blvd., #555
Anchorage, AK 99503
(907) 561–5322 Fax (907) 561–0334

Arizona
Arizona Hospice Organization
P.O. Box 1686
Tempe, AZ 85280–1686
(602) 752–3523 Fax (602) 752–3523

Arkansas
Arkansas State Hospice Association
c/o Hospice of the Ozarks
701 Burnett Dr.
Mountain Home, AR 72653
(501) 424–1790 Fax (501) 424–1660

California
California State Hospice Association
2023 N St., Ste. 205
P.O. Box 160087
Sacramento, CA 95816
(916) 441–3770 Fax (916) 441–4720

Colorado
Colorado State Hospice Organization
c/o Hospice of Peace
1620 Meade St.
Denver, CO 80204
(303) 575–8393 Fax (303) 575–8390

Connecticut
Hospice Council of Connecticut
60 Lorraine St.
Hartford, CT 06105
(860) 233–2222

Delaware
Delaware Hospice, Inc
Clayton Bldg.
3515 Silverside Rd., Ste. 100
Wilmington, DE 19810
(302) 478–5707 Fax (302) 479–2586

District of Columbia
Hospice Council of Metro Washington
c/o Hospice of Northern Virginia
6400 Arlington Blvd., Ste. 1000
Falls Church, VA 22042
(703) 534–7070 Fax (703) 538–2163

Florida
Florida Hospices, Inc.
c/o Hospice of North Central Florida
3615 S.W. 13th St.
P.O. Box 15235
Gainesville, FL 32604
(904) 378–2121 Fax (904) 378–4111

Georgia
Georgia Hospice Organization
c/o Kennestone Regional Hospice
P.O. Box 1208
Marietta, GA 30061–9975
(770) 793–7370 Fax (770) 793–7925

Hawaii
Hawaii State Hospice Network
c/o Hospice Hawaii
445 Seaside, Ste. 604
Honolulu, HI 96815–2676
(808) 924–9255 Fax (808) 922–9161

Idaho
Idaho Hospice Organization
c/o Hospice of the Wood Valley
P.O. Box 4320
Ketchum, ID 83340–4320
(208) 726–8464 Fax (208) 726–1074

Illinois
Illinois State Hospice Organization
1525 E. 53rd St., Ste. 720
Chicago, IL 60615
(312) 324–8844 Fax (312) 324–8247

Indiana
Indiana Association of Hospices
2142 W. 86th St.
Indianapolis, IN 46260
(317) 338–4716 Fax (317) 338–4757

Iowa
Iowa Hospice Organization
4815 University Ave., Ste. 2
Des Moines, IA 50311
(515) 277–0281 Fax (515) 277–0284

Kansas
Association of Kansas Hospices
1901 University
Wichita, KS 67213–3325
(316) 263–6380 Fax (316) 263–6542

Kentucky
Kentucky Association of Hospices
c/o Community Hospice
1538 Central Ave.
Ashland, KY 41101
(606) 329–1890 Fax (606) 329–0018

Louisiana
Louisiana Hospice Organization
c/o Hospice of South Louisiana
210 Mystic Blvd.
Houma, LA 70360–2762
(504) 851–4273 Fax (504) 872–6543

Maine
Maine Hospice Council
16 Winthrop St.
Augusta, ME 04330
(207) 626–0651 Fax (207) 626–0651

Maryland
Hospice Network of Maryland
5820 Southwestern Blvd.
Baltimore, MD 21227
(410) 242–1975 Fax (410) 247–4426

Massachusetts
Hospice Federation of Massachusetts
1420 Providence Hwy., Ste. 216
Norwood, MA 02062
(617) 255–7077 Fax (617) 255–7078

Michigan
Michigan Hospice Organization
7201 W. Saginaw Hwy., Ste. 312
Lansing, MI 48917
(517) 886–6667 Fax (517) 886–6737

Minnesota
Minnesota Hospice Organization
Iris Park Place, Ste. 36
1885 University Ave W.
St. Paul, MN 55104–3403
(612) 659–0423 Fax (612) 659–9126

Mississippi
Mississippi Hospice Organization
c/o Hospice of Central Mississippi
2600 Insurance Center Dr., Ste. B120
Jackson, MS 39216
(601) 336–9881 Fax (601) 981–0150

Missouri
Missouri Hospice Organization
c/o Kansas City Hospice
1625 W. 92nd St.
Kansas City, MO 64114
(816) 363–2600 Fax (816) 523–0068

Montana
Montana Hospice Organization
c/o Gateway Hospice
504 S. 13th St.
Livingston, MT 59047
(406) 222–5030 Fax (406) 222–5099

Nebraska
Nebraska Hospice Association
R.R. 1, Box 66
Palmer, NE 68864
(308) 894–5400 Fax (308) 384–1239

Nevada
Hospice Association of Nevada
c/o Family Home Hospice
P.O. Box 15645
Las Vegas, NV 89114–5645
(702) 383–0887 Fax (702) 383–1173

New Hampshire
New Hampshire Hospice Organization
P.O. Box 638
Concord, NH 03302–0638
(800) 639–8594 Fax (802) 295–3163

New Jersey
New Jersey Hospice Organization
175 Glenside Ave.
Scotch Plains, NJ 07076
(908) 233–0060 Fax (908) 233–1630

New Mexico
New Mexico Hospice Organization
c/o GRMC Hospice
1313 E. 32nd St.
Silver City, NM 88061
(505) 388–2273 Fax (505) 388–1448

New York
New York State Hospice Association
21 Aviation Rd., Ste. 9
Albany, NY 12205
(518) 446–1483 Fax (518) 446–1484

North Carolina
Hospice for the Carolinas
400 Oberlin Rd., Ste. 300
Raleigh, NC 27605
(919) 829–9588 Fax (919) 829–1383

North Dakota
North Dakota Hospice Organization
c/o United Hospice
1200 S. Columbia Rd.
Grand Forks, ND 58206
(701) 780–5258

Ohio
Ohio Hospice Organization
2400 Briggs Rd.
Columbus, OH 43223
(614) 274–9513 Fax (614) 274–6357

Oklahoma
Oklahoma State Hospice Association
c/o Hospice of Green Country
3010 S. Harvard, Ste. 110
Tulsa, OK 74114
(918) 747–2273 Fax (918) 747–2573

Oregon
Oregon Hospice Association
P.O. Box 10796
Portland, OR 97210
(503) 228–2104 Fax (503) 222–4907

Pennsylvania
Pennsylvania Hospice Network
128 State St., Ste. 200
P.O. Box 60636,
Harrisburg, PA 17106–0636
(717) 230–9993 Fax (717) 230–9997

Puerto Rico
Puerto Rico Home Health & Hospice Association
P.O. Box 192152
San Juan, PR 00919–2152
(809) 743–1121

Rhode Island
Rhode Island State Hospice Organization
c/o Hospice of VNS
14 Woodruff Ave.
Narragansett, RI 02882
(401) 788–2052 Fax (401) 788–2064

South Carolina
Hospice for the Carolinas
241 Lake Summit Court
Chapin, SC 29036
(919) 829–9588 Fax (919) 829–1383

South Dakota
South Dakota Hospice Organization
c/o Mitchell Community Hospice
525 N. Foster
Mitchell, SD 57301
(605) 995–2441 Fax (605) 995–2268

Tennessee
Tennessee Hospice Organization
P.O. Box 24685
Nashville, TN 37202
(615) 327–1085

Texas
Texas Hospice Organization
3724 Jefferson #318
Austin, TX 78731
(512) 454–1247 Fax (512) 454–1248

Utah
Utah Hospice Organization
c/o Health Watch Hospice
1384 State St.
Pleasant Grove, UT 84062
(801) 785–8848 Fax (801) 785–0821

Vermont
Hospice Council of Vermont
52 State St.
Montpelier, VT 05602
(802) 229–0579

Virginia
Virginia Association for Hospice
P.O. Box 34765
Richmond, VA 23234
(804) 743–7644 Fax (804) 743–7941

Washington
Washington State Hospice Organization
908 W. Bellwood Dr., Ste. 100
Spokane, WA 99218
(509) 466–1064 Fax (509) 466–1421

West Virginia
Hospice Council of West Virginia
P.O. Box 229
Kingwood, WV 26537
(304) 329–1161 Fax (304) 329–3285

Wisconsin
Hospice Organization of Wisconsin
P.O. Box 366
Whitewater, WI 53190
(414) 473–7847 Fax (414) 473–7867

Wyoming
Wyoming Hospice Organization
317 W. 14th St.
Casper, WY 82601–4203
(307) 473–7411 Fax (307) 473–8954

References

Abrams, D., et al. "AIDS: Caring for the Dying Patient." *Patient Care* 23, no. 19 (1989): 23–36.

Altman, L. "AIDS Tests of Health Workers Called Unnecessary." *New York Times*, 23 February 1991, p. 9.

Anderson, H., and P. MacElveen-Hoehn. "Gay Clients with AIDS: New Challenges for Hospice Programs." *Hospice Journal* 4 (1988): 38–39.

Andrulis, D., et al. "The Provision and Financing of Medical Care for AIDS Patients in the U.S. Public and Private Teaching Hospitals." *Journal of the American Medical Association* 258, no. 10 (1987): 1343–46.

Arno, P. "The Nonprofit Sector's Response to the AIDS Epidemic: Community-Based Services in San Francisco." *American Journal of Public Health* 76, no. 11 (1986): 1325–30.

Benjamin, A. "Long-term Care and AIDS: Perspectives from Experience with the Elderly." *Milbank Quarterly* 66, no. 3 (1988): 415–43.

Benjamin, B., M. Young, and C. Wallis. "Mortality of Widowers." *Lancet* 2 (1963): 454–56.

Beresford, L. "Alternative Outpatient Settings of Care for People with AIDS." *Quarterly Review Bulletin* 1 (1989): 9–16.

Berger, R. "Cost of AIDS Patients in Maryland." *Maryland State Medical Journal* 34 (1986): 1173.

Birnbaum, H., and D. Kidder. "What Does Hospice Cost?" *American Journal of Public Health* 74 (1992): 689–97.

Bischoff, W. "A Cost Allocation Model for Hospice." *Nursing Management* 24, no. 12 (1993): 38–41.

Bloom, B., and P. Kissick. "Home and Hospital Cost of Terminal Illness." *Medical Care* 18, no. 5 (n.d.): 560–64.

Bluebond-Langer, M. *The Private World of Dying Children.* Princeton, N.J.: Princeton University Press, 1978.

Bowlby, J. "Processes of Mourning." *International Journal of Psychoanalysis* 44 (1961): 317.

Buckingham, R. *Care of the Dying Child: A Practical Guide for Those Who Help Others.* New York: Continuum, 1990.

Buckingham, R., and D. Lupu. "A Comparative Study of Hospice Services in the United States." *American Journal of Public Health* 72 (1982): 455.

Bulkin, W., and H. Lukashok, "Rx for Dying: The Case for Hospice." *New England Journal of Medicine* 318, no. 6 (1988): 316–78.

Chinn, P. *Child Health Maintenance.* St. Louis, Mo.: C.V. Mosby, 1974.

Clark, C., et al. "Hospice Care: A Model for Caring for the Persons with AIDS." *Nursing Clinics of North America* 23 (1988): 851–62.

Clayton, P., J. Halikes, and W. Maurice. "The Bereavement of the Widowed." *Diseases of the Nervous System* 32 (1971): 597–604.

Cohen, K. *Hospice, Prescription of Terminal Care.* Germantown, Md.: Aspen Systems Corporation, 1979.

Corles, I., and M. Pittman-Lindeman. *AIDS Principles, Practice, and Politics.* New York: Hemisphere Publishing Corporation, 1989.

Corr, C. and D. Corr. *Hospice Care: Principles and Practice.* New York: Springer Publishing Company, 1983.

Dunton, D. "The Child's Concept of Death." In *Loss and Grief: Psychological Management in Medical Practice,* ed. B. Schoenberg. New York: Columbia University Press, 1970.

Durham, J., and F. Cohen. *The Person with AIDS.* New York: Springer Publishing Company, 1987.

"The Epidemiology of AIDS in the U.S." *Scientific American* 259 (n.d.): 72–81.

Feifel, H. "Perception of Death." *Annals of the New York Academy of Science* 164 (1969): 669.

———. *New Meanings of Death.* New York: McGraw-Hill, 1977.

Friedland, G. "Clinical Care in the AIDS Epidemic." *Daedalus* 118 (1989): 67–78.

Friedman, S., et al. "Behavioral Observations of Parents Anticipating the Death of a Child." In *Counseling Par-*

ents of the Ill and the Handicapped, ed. R. Nolan. Springfield, Ill.: Charles Thomas, 1971.

Friedman, S. B. "Behavioral Observations of Parents Anticipating the Death of a Child." *Pediatrics* 32, no. 3 (1963).

Furman, E. *A Child's Parent Dies.* New Haven, Conn.: Yale University Press, 1974.

Glaser, B., and A. Strauss. *Awareness of Dying.* Chicago: Aldine de Gruyter, 1965.

Green, J., et al. "Projecting the Impact of AIDS on Hospitals." *Health Affairs* 6, no. 3 (1987): 19–31.

Green, M. "Care of the Child with a Long-term, Life-Threatening Illness: Some Principles of Management." *Pediatrics* 39, no. 3 (1967).

Grollman, E. *Concerning Death: A Practical Guide for the Living.* Boston: Beacon Press, 1974.

"Guidelines for the Protection of Health Care Workers in Caring for Persons Who Have Some form of HTLV-III/LAV Infection." *New York Journal of Medicine* 86, no. 11 (n.d.): 587–91.

Gut, E. "Some Aspects of Adult Mourning." *Omega* 5 (1974): 335.

Gyulay, J. E. *The Dying Child.* New York: McGraw-Hill/Blakiston, 1978.

Hardy, A. M., et al. "The Economic Impact of the First 10,000 Cases of Acquired Immunodeficiency Syndrome in the United States." *Journal of the American Medical Association* 255, no. 2 (1986): 19–31.

Haseltine, W. "Prospects for the Medical Control of the AIDS Epidemic." *Daedalus* 118 (1989): 14.

Hendin, D. *Death as a Fact of Life.* New York: Norton, 1973.

Hollingsworth, C., and R. Pasnau. *The Family in Mourning: A Guide for Health Professionals.* New York: Grune & Stratton, 1977.

Howell, E. "The Role of Community-Based Organizations in Responding to the AIDS Epidemic: Examples from the HRSA Service Demonstration." *Journal of Public Health Policy* 12, no. 2 (1991): 165–73.

"Human Immunodeficiency Virus Infections in Children: Public Health and Policy Issues." *Pediatric Infectious Disease Journal* 6 (1987): 113–16.

Iglehart, J., et al. "The Socioeconomic Impact of AIDS on Health Care Systems." *Health Affairs* 6, no. 3 (1987): 137–47.

Institute of Medicine "Care of Persons Infected with HIV." In *Confronting AIDS: Update 1988.* Washington, D.C.: National Academy Press, 1988.

Johnson, J. *AIDS: An Overview of Issues* (CRS Report No. 1B87150). Washington, D.C.: Library of Congress, 1991.

Jones, A. "Hospices and Homecare Agencies: Data from the 1991 National Health Provider Inventory (NHPI). Division of Health Care Statistics." *Advance Data* 257 (November 1994): 1–7.

Kalish, R. *Death, Grief, and Caring Relationships.* Pacific Grove, Calif.: Brooks, Cole Publishing Company, 1981.

Kawata, P., and J. Andriote. "NAN—A National Voice for Community-Based Services for Persons with AIDS." *Public Health Reports* 103, no. 3 (1988): 299–304.

Kimmel, D. *Adulthood and Aging.* New York: Wiley, 1974.

Kizer, K., et al. *An Updated Quantitive Analysis of AIDS in California.* Sacramento: California Department of Health Services, n.d.

Koocher, G. P. "Talking with Children about Death." *American Journal of Orthopsychiatry* 44, no. 3 (1974): 410.

Kübler-Ross, E. *On Death and Dying*. New York: Macmillan, 1969.

Lack, S., and R. Buckingham. *First American Hospice: Three Years of Home Care*. New Haven, Conn.: Hospice, Inc., 1978.

Landers, S., and G. Seage. "Medical Care of AIDS in New England: Costs and Implications." In *The AIDS Epidemic: Private Rights and Public Interest*, ed. P. O'Malley. Boston: Beacon Press, 1989.

Lattanzi-Licht, and S. Conner. "Care of the Dying: The Hospice Approach." In *Dying: Facing the Facts*, eds. H. Wass and R. Neimeyer. Washington, D.C.: Taylor & Francis, 1995.

Librach, S. "Who's in Control? What's in a Family?" *Journal of Palliative Care* 4, no. 1 (1988): 1–12.

Mansell, P. "AIDS: Home, Ambulatory, and Palliative Care." *Journal of Palliative Care* 4 (1988): 31–32.

Martin, J. "Ensuring Quality Hospice Care for the Person with AIDS." *Quality Review Bulletin* 10 (1986): 353–58.

———. "Hospice and Home Care for Persons with AIDS/ARC." *Death Studies* 12 (1988): 468–69.

Martinson, I. A. "Home Care for Children Dying of Cancer." *Pediatrics* 62, no. 1 (1978): 108.

McCaffery, M. "Pain Management: Nurses Lead the Way to New Priorities." *American Journal of Nursing* 90 (1990): 45–46.

McKell, D. *Hospice Care: A New Concept for the Care of the Terminally Ill and Their Families*. Workshop at UCLA Extension, Los Angeles, April 1978.

Mor, V. *Hospice Care Systems: Structure, Process Costs,*

and Outcome. New York: Springer Publishing Company, 1987.

Mor, V., and D. Kidder. "Cost Savings in Hospice: Final Results of the National Hospice Study." *Health Services Research* 20, no. 4 (1988): 407–22.

Moss, V. "The Mildmay Approach." *Journal of Palliative Care* 4 (1988): 105.

National Association for Home Care. "NAHC 1995 Legislative Reports." *Blueprints for Action* (February 1995): 9–69.

O'Connor, J., et al. "Does Care Exclude Cure in Palliative Care?" *Journal of Palliative Care* 2 (1986): 11–15.

Palmer, G. "Singles World." In *Alone and Surviving,* ed. R. Lindsay. New York: Walker, 1977.

Parkes, C. *Bereavement: Studies of Grief in Adult Life.* New York: International University Free Press, 1972.

———. "Recent Bereavement as a Cause of Mental Illness." *British Journal of Psychiatry* 110 (1964): 198–204.

Parkes, C., and R. Brown. "Health after Bereavement: A Controlled Study of Young Boston Widows and Widowers." *Psychosomatic Medicine* 34 (1972): 449–60.

Pike, D. *Life Is Victorious: How to Grow through Grief.* New York: Simon, and Schuster, 1976.

Powazek, M. "Emotional Reactions of Children to Isolation in a Cancer Hospital." *Journal of Pediatrics* 92, no. 5 (1978): 836.

"Pregnancies Resulting in Infants with Acquired Immunodeficiency Syndrome or AIDS-Related Complex: Follow-up of Mothers, Children, Subsequently Born Siblings." *Obstetrics & Gynecology* 69 (July/August 1988): 285–91.

"Quarterly Report to the Domestic Policy Council on the Prevalence and Rate of Spread of HIV and AIDS in the United States." *Journal of American Medical Association* 259, no. 18 (1988): 2657–61.

Rees, D, and S. Lutkins. "Mortality of Bereavement." *British Medical Journal* (October 1967).

Rhymes, J. "Hospice Care in America." *Journal of the American Medical Association* 264, no. 3 (1990): 369–72.

Roper, W., and W. Winkenwerder. "Making Fair Decisions about Financing Care for Persons with AIDS. *Public Health Reports* 103, no. 3 (n.d.): 305–308.

Rothenberg, R., et al. "Survival with the Acquired Immunodeficiency Syndrome: Experience with 5,833 Cases in New York City." *New England Journal of Medicine* 317, no. 21 (1987): 1297–1302.

Samaniego, L. R. "Exploring the Physically Ill Child's Self-Perceptions and the Mother's Perceptions of Her Child's Needs." *Clinical Pediatrics* 19, no. 2 (1977): 157.

Schiff, H. *The Bereaved Parent.* New York: Penguin Books, 1978.

Schoefferman, J. "Care of the AIDS Patient." *Death Studies* 12 (1988): 446.

Schowelter, J. "Parent's Death and Childhood Bereavement." In *Bereavement: It's Psychological Aspects,* ed. B. Schoenberg. New York: Columbia University Press, 1975.

Scitovsky, A. "Studying the Cost of HIV-Related Illnesses: Reflections of a Moving Target." *Millbank Quarterly* 67, no. 2 (1989): 318–46.

Scitovsky, A., M. Kline, and P. Lee. "Medical Care Costs

of Patients with AIDS in San Francisco." *Journal of the American Medical Association* 256, no. 22 (1986): 3103–3106.

Scitovsky, A., and D. Rice. "Estimates of the Direct and Indirect Costs of Acquired Immunodeficiency Syndrome in the United States, 1985, 1986, and 1991." *Public Health Reports* 102, no. 1 (1987): 5–17, 3102–3106.

Seage, G., et al. "Medical Care Costs of AIDS in Massachusetts." *Journal of the American Medical Association* 256, no. 22 (1986): 3106–3109.

——. "Effect of Changing Patterns of Care and Duration of Survival on the Cost of Treating the Acquired Immunodeficiency Syndrome (AIDS)." *American Journal of Public Health* 80, no. 7 (1990): 835–39.

Shephard, D. "Terminal Care: Towards an Ideal." *Canadian Medical Association Journal* 115 (1976): 97–98.

——. "Principles and Practice of Palliative Care." *Canadian Medical Association Journal* 116 (1977): 522–26.

Shoor, M., and M. Speed. "Delinquency as a Manifestation of the Mourning Process." *Psychiatric Quarterly* 37 (1963).

Sisk, J. "The Cost of AIDS: A Review of the Estimates." *Health Affairs* 6, no. 2 (1987): 5–20.

Stephany, T. "AIDS and the Hospice Nurse." *Home Health Nurse* 8, no. 2 (1990): 141–54.

Stoddard, S. *The Hospice Movement.* New York: Stein & Day, 1978.

Tsoukas, C. "The Dying Leper Syndrome." *Journal of Palliative Care* 4 (1988): 13–14.

"Update on HIV Infection: Pediatric Aspects." *Maryland Medical Journal* 36, no. 1 (n.d.): 37–39.

U.S. Department of Health and Human Services, Centers for Disease Control. "Recommendations for Prevention of HIV Transmission in Health Care Settings." *Morbidity and Mortality Weekly Report* 36, no. 2S (1987): 15-S.

———. "Review of the CDC Surveillances Case Definition for Acquired Immunodeficiency Syndrome." *Morbidity and Mortality Weekly Report* (Suppl.) 36, no. lS (1987): 15.

Worden, J. *Grief Counseling and Grief Therapy.* New York: Springer Publishing Company, 1982.

World Health Organization. *Bridging the Gaps: 1995 World Health Report.* Geneva: World Health Organization, 1995.

Zimmerman, J. *Hospice: Complete Care for the Terminally Ill.* Baltimore and Munich: Urban and Schwarzenberg, 1986.